MEDICAL MARIJUANA
CHANGING TIMES III

Contents

3   Information: Additional Info

❖   **Definitions**

I   Information: Medicinal Marijuana

PATIENT SUFFERING

Many patients suffering from diseases also suffer from side effects of their treatments, 75 percent of New York voters support legalizing medical marijuana to help seriously ill patients. The Assembly has been fighting over medical marijuana bills for eight years now. Currently 11 states allow marijuana for medical use, Arizona, California, Colorado, Alaska, Hawaii, Maine, Montana, Nevada, Vermont, Oregon, Rhode Island and Washington. In 2005 the Supreme Court ruled that the Federal Government right to prosecute medical marijuana users over rides the states right to help people with their illnesses. There is a conflict between the states and the Federal Government over medical marijuana. The Federal Government should not prosecute medical marijuana patients that are taking medical marijuana in compliance with state laws. In the 1980's when the states and Federal Government first started realizing the benefits of medical to help patients, the National Institute of Drug Abuse provided marijuana to the New York State Department of Health for a study. The study found that 78 percent of 56 patients who smoked the state sponsored marijuana that had chemotherapy induced nausea and appetite loss showed that the marijuana increased appetite and help with the nausea.

The test patients maintain or increased their body weight. Many of the test patients opted for medical marijuana, after all the other anti-nausea medications were no longer effective. One would think since the study had positive results that it would be made available for medical patients who are suffering from chronic pain and other illnesses that have exhausted all other medicines to treat their illness. There are now 13 states that have laws allowing therapeutic research programs with Federal cooperation, and 10 states, including New York, have symbolic laws which would allow patients to possess prescription Medical Marijuana if the Federal law were ever to be changed.

CURE?

Medical Marijuana is not a cure but an aid in treatment for many different illnesses. Medical Marijuana has several effects, such as a mild mind and body relaxer, a pick me up type of feeling good, appetite inducer, Regarding recreation drugs and alcohol I always ask the question, why do people take drugs? The answer is always the same, to feel better or feel good. So that means they don't feel well and want to feel better. Many people take drugs and alcohol recreationally and think they need to have it to have a good time. Medical Marijuana is not for recreational purposes. Its purpose serves a need that helps many people with their real illnesses and beneficial. Medicinal plants and health disorders;. The organizations of the complex organs, cells, and tissues in the human body have differing function in sink and properly. When the bodies network are not working properly or missing because of viruses, fungi, burns, parasites infections, bacteria, inherited gene defects, . Health disorders are treated in many ways if the causes are known. Many health disorders are complex that only symptomatic treatments are used. Synthetic medicines are available for health disorders which are powerful and exhibit a lot of undesired side effects. Medicines derived from plants are usually less specific, and can affect more than one molecular area which can be helpful in complex health disorders.

For thousands of years in Asia herbal healers have been prescribing marijuana for treatments. In China the Chinese herbal healers have it down to an art of accuracy in prescribing the correct herbal medicine for specific illnesses, as well in Myanmar, Thailand, Vietnam, and India. An elderly couple named Wo and Mayling Lee of Nanning China lived on their farm raising chickens and growing vegetables. It came to light that Mr. Lee had arthritis in his hands which prevented him from maintaining his farm work. After trying different doctors and medications with no positive results, Mrs. Lee began to do more work around the farm to take up the slack for her husband but that soon began to take its toll on her. The stress and pressure of her husband illness and the extra work drove her into depression. Mrs. Lee began drinking Green tea and marijuana in the late afternoons which was having a positive effect on her stress and depression. It helped her cope with her situation. Mr. Lee would smoke the marijuana in a handmade pipe saying that it helped the discomfort in his hands. In Vietnam the hemp plants which is marijuana is used for many different purposes from rope, clothes, brooms, baskets, and medicine combinations. In most of the villages the people relied on what they grow and utilizing what their environment offers. Marijuana has been used all over the world for thousands of years for medical use.

HERBAL HEALERS

In 800 BC the Aztec and native people had herbal healers that prescribed marijuana in different forms according to the ailment and age of the patient. The herbal healers used their whole world as their pharmacy and plants as their medicines. The herb was made in a liquid form for the young or eaten and was dried like tobacco for smoking by the elderly. In these time periods before modern medicines and the advent of doctors there were shamans, wizards, witches, witchdoctors, herbal healers, and sorcerers. Herbal healers is almost a lost art. The knowledge of what herbs are prescribed to treat a specific ailment was handed down from generation to generation. Even in today's time in South America there are herbal healers. There are many different types and strains of marijuana plants that have different potency an ideal tropical climate for thousands of years. Before the age of modern medicines people were more dependent upon natural Earth medicines. Unlike today more people in the past used the Earth's natural bounty of foods, minerals, herbs, est., for good health. Herbal medications have been used for thousands of years in the past and will be used in the future for as long as humans inhabit this planet. Some jungles in South America are considered natures pharmacy because of all the many natural plants and products that era utilized by man. The American Indians are another example of a people that lived off of the land and nature's bounty. There were many different tribes, some would migrate annually from North to South. Some would migrate constantly by following the Buffalo herds. Others would not migrate and stay in one location and relocate only when necessary. The Indians that lived in the forest were called forest people. These

Indians lived totally off of the land by growing food, fishing, hunting, and collecting anything that could have some use. The elderly woman would pass down from generation to the next generation the knowledge of what plants were useful and which plants are not. In the year of 1350 in North America there lived a people known as the Black Foot tribes. It was believed that the Black Foot people numbers ranged from 50 thousand to several hundred thousand. Living in separate Craws or tribes that are separated by land distances each had its own tribal council and chief. The tribal leader would stay in contact with each other by way of using smoke signals or foot messengers. In the tribal council were the wisest elder men of the tribe. These men and their chief made all important policy regarding the tribe. Keep in mind that there were dozens of tribes each having a tribal council of wise men. In most cases one of the council men was also the tribal witch doctor. The itch doctor or the other name was medicine man would be the tribal doctor and spiritual leader of the tribe that he lived with. The medicine man would use many different herbs including marijuana to treat many different illnesses. The Black Foot elderly women past down from generation to generation the knowledge of the uses herbs, plants, and roots.

THE TRIBES OF AMERICA

The tribes would migrate from North to South in the winter and from the South to the North in the summer time. The men were hunters and fisherman and the women took care of the family unit and its needs. The Black Foot Indians were a proud and strong people especially the women. It would come to pass in the 1700's the Black Foot Indians women's name would change to the walking women, because of the new times of having to migrate on a constant basis. During this time period the Back Foot braves preferred death over being forced to an Indian reservation. Freedom and the land is all he knew and without it he preferred death were as the Black Foot woman would learn how to adapt to their situation. Most of the knowledge of herbal medicines was lost for many years and some knowledge was lost forever. Before the 1700's the medicine man had a great deal of power and influence over his location and tribe. His duties were medical, spiritual, and cancelling for his tribe. In order to have the trust and confidence of the tribal members, he would have to be knowledgeable with his duties to the tribe. The medicine man would know about all the plants, herbs, and natures natural medicines. In many cases the medicine man would use a combination of plants and medicines and herbs that included marijuana to treat many different illnesses. Herbal and plant medicines have been used for thousands of years for the treatment of illnesses all over the world. Human beings have utilized herbal medicines since the beginning of man kink and will continue to use herbal medicines for as long as the earth yields it. In the 15th and 16th century in Africa there were many tribes like the Nudies, Musonis, Unganase, Zulu, Owabie, ext.. These tribes all have had a witch doctor, elder healer whose job was to help the physical and mental and spiritual needs of their people. They would utilize all of nature's bounty in their efforts to help their people. They would use all types of combinations of herbs for different treatments of illnesses including marijuana. Herbal medicine combinations have been past down from generation to generation for hundreds of years. Even before man learned how to forge metal, there were herbal healers taking care of the needs of their people. It was found that in a ancient burial site said to be thousands of years old. Archeologist found marijuana seeds that had petrified. Suggesting that marijuana was used in conjunction with a burial ceremony or ritual. Marijuana was also used for spiritual purposes as well as medical purposes. 500 years ago there were herbal healers in the 14th century Europe one of which was Michel Nostradamus who was not only known for his predictions but for his medical knowledge in healing others. During this time period the people were afflicted with wide spread contagious disease associated with a high death rate. The disease was called the Black Plague and epidemic disease with high mortality that swept through Europe during the 14th century. As a young man M. Nostradamus would help treat people with this fatal disease with medicines, herbs, and good clean practices. Nostradamus experimented with different herbs including marijuana. In his travels to other counties in search of medicinal herbs from 1521 to 1529. During this time period there were no laws pertaining to the use of any of the herbal medicines for better health. Nostradamus was an expert with herbal medicines. Back

5

at that time all herbal healers used marijuana at one time or any other to treat numerous types of illnesses, mental and physical. In changing times modern man will to or realize the medical benefits of marijuana as was realized in man's past.

The Amazon River and The Rain Forest tribes. There are a few Amazonian tribes that have had no contact with the outside world. These tribes lived totally independent and away from any other tribes or people. These tribes would stay hidden from others and have no contact with the outside world or others. These tribes led a very simple life, off of nature. These lost tribes chose to stay in solitude living off the land and nature for many generations. Utilizing everything in their forest. Hunting, fishing, and harvesting plants for their medical uses including marijuana. It was found that these tribes that had no contact with the outside world were all in all healthier and lived longer due to their isolation from civilization. The pressure of one's daily life style of the average modern person is many times greater than a forest Indian's life style. Daily life in the modern world is much more stressful and wearing on a person that takes its toll. These forest tribes were disease free and were physically fit. Even at the age of 50 to 60 years old. Any one member of ether of these tribes would find it almost impossible to adapt to modern man's life style as well as a modern man would find it very hard to adapt to a tribal member's life style. They also used the hemp plant fibers to make all sizes of ropes and heavy clothes. Some questions we all ask like why people that don't have any medical illnesses take marijuana. Some will say, to have a good time or make them relaxed. Or to divert their minds from their daily problems for a short time. Some will say they take it to feel better. To feel better from what? The daily mental stresses of life or something else? Tens of thousands of people are taking marijuana coast to coast and half will say to get high and the other half will say to feel better. To feel better infers that one is not feeling well and needs to feel m better. The term (get high) infers that one is feeling the opposite which is low. The term feeling low can be interpreted as a form and degree of depression. Many people will take prescription medications, drink alcohol or take marijuana for all the wrong reasons. And yet prescription medications or drinking alcohol can be more addictive and more harmful than medical marijuana. Still medical marijuana is still illegal in most States but with changing times and advancement in the future the obsolete laws of the past will be revised. With changing times in the future the States and Government will come to the realization that they will benefit from regulating the use of medical marijuana for patients that have permits. Eventually in the near future the State and Federal Government will regulate its medical use through the Bureau of Alcohol, Tobacco, and Firearms.

THE CONCEPT: MEDICINAL MARIJUANA

The term medical marijuana is relativity new and yet marijuana has been used for medical purpose for thousands of years. Even though these modern times we live in, the 21 century a few of today's laws need to be repealed or amended regarding medical marijuana. One would think that the powers that be or certain special interest groups, powerful people or companies do not want the legalization of medical marijuana because of their financial reasons. There are a few States that have programs pertaining to medical marijuana available. Medical marijuana is grown in laboratories, Government sponsored farms which set aside a small piece of land to grow it. Small amounts of medical marijuana are shipped and picked up with a doctor's prescription and medical identification by the patient. In some areas where there is legalization of medical marijuana the patient will grow medical marijuana on their own property in small amounts for medical use. Most doctors will not prescribe medical marijuana because of the stigmatism and all the other modern medicines on the market. There's hardly any information pertaining to it. One saving grace is that all things change in time as will man and woman advance in to the future. The laws will change to accommodate the new times.

When these new changes are made to the laws pertaining to medical marijuana it is predicted that there will be special licenses for the sale of medical marijuana with a doctor's prescription in pharmacy's or clinics. All the patients would have a medical marijuana I.D. permit, which would enable them to purchase or grow marijuana in small amounts. In the pharmacies or clinics medical marijuana would be sold in pill form or natural organic form.

7

There will be different potencies according to the strength of THC. The doctor would prescribe the correct amount to treat specific illnesses. Eventually pharmacies and clinics will have different grades and types of medical marijuana available with prescription only. Patients will have the freedom to grow marijuana in small amounts inside their homes or outside their homes. Some patients will require less potent medical marijuana for their specific illness and some patients will require more potent marijuana to treat their illness. As time goes on the accuracy will increase greatly in rating potency, grade and type of marijuana and have a nationwide rating system in place. With these systems in place doctors from coast to coast would be able to refer to for their patients. Naturally the Government and State would have control with taxing and regulate medical marijuana in the some fashion that they have taxes on cigarettes and drinking alcohol. With taxing medical marijuana the Government and State would receive great amount of money for their coppers.

MEDICAL MARIJUANA TREATABLE ILLNESSES

A brief list of medical illnesses currently treated with medicinal marijuana:

Adult ADD, Agitated Depression, AIDS Disease, Alcoholism, Anger Management, Anorexia Nervosa, Ankylosing Spondylitis, Appetite Loss, Arthritis, Alzheimer's Disease, Bipolar Disorder, Bronzed Diabetes, Bulimia Nervosa, Bursitis, Cancer Disease, Carpal Tunnel Syndrome, Collagen Disease, Chronic Disease, Crohn's Disease, Depression, Dermatomyositis Disease, Diabetes Digestive System, Elevated Stress, Fibrocystic Breast Disease, Fibromyalgia, Glaucoma, GLIMA, Gout, Hemochromatosis, Herniated Disk, Hyperthyroidism, Insomnia, Kaposi's Sarcoma, Leukemia, Lou Gehrig's Disease (ALS), Lupus Disease, Mania, Meningitis Virus, Mensal Cramps, Mood Swings, Muscular Rheumatism, Multiple Sclerosis (MS), Malaria, Neoplasm, Neurasthenia, Osteoarthritis, Osteoporosis, Panic Disorder, Personality Neurosis Disorder, Phobias, Premenstrual Syndrome, Polymyositis, Polymyalgia Rheumatic, Post Traumatic Stress Disorder, Pseudo gout, Psoriatic Arthritis, Reiter's Syndrome, Rheumatoid Arthritis, Sciatica Pain, Scoliosis, Scleroderma,

Sickle Cell Anemia, Spondylus Thyropathy, Soft tissue Rheumatism, Jorgen's Syndrome, Stiff man Syndrome, Stress, TB, Tendinitis, Tennis Elbow, Temporomandibular Joint Syndrome.

OTHER HERBS AND SPICES TO TREAT ILLNESSES

American Ginseng: action notion Lungs, Spleen, Liver, Energies. Good for general weakness, poor immunity, stomach pain. Basil: helps the stomach. Chili Pepper: helps blood circulation. Clinnam Bark: helps the Kidney, Spleen, Liver, good for weakness, poor circulation,. Cloves: helps Liver, Spleen, good for heavy menstruation. Lavender: good for nervous disorder. St. John's Wort: good for depression,. Gin Kgo Biloba: good for mood swings, Dementia, low stamina,. Yellow Jasmine: good for Anxiety, headaches. A FEW ILLNESSES and HERBS and SPICES taken to treat them: Alcohol abuse-Kudzuvine (PUERARIA IOBATA). Hypertension, Anxiety, Insomnia, Indian Snakeroot (Rauvollia serpentine). For Strength and endurance-Roseroot, Arctic root, (Rhodioda rosea). High blood pressure, Rue herb of grace (Ruta graveolens). X-Alcohol treatment, Hypnotic sedative, moods, Anxiety. Stress. Sciaticum (Sorbus aucuparia) is taken for Diabetes, Kidney disorder, Arthritis and many other illnesses. Cat's Claw is taken for AIDS, Herpes, Cancer, Diabetes, Arthritis. There are many, many more Herbs and Spices that have been taken throughout the ages.

CIVILIZATIONS USING PLANTS

Human civilization always used plants for its needs. Even before man started living in a house and was living in a cave, he would use any and all natures plants to utilize its benefits. Marijuana in conjunction with other herbs has been taken ever since humans became civilized and even before that. Marijuana has been used in many medicines in conjunction with other herbs by ancient peoples in many parts of the world. It had been used in many religious rituals and even in love passions. Ancient Egypt, Samarian, The Nazca People, The Mayans, Ancient African Tribes, The Aztec People, and many more people throughout time. Ancient American Indians would hold strange tribal traditions and had a constant presence of religious activities in daily life and a habit of participation in religious activities. Sometimes some of the Indians would take Peyote from the Peyote Plant, marijuana, Loco Weed for religious rituals and ceremony. Elderly people in the tribes would take marijuana for numerous illnesses, from back aces to Arthritis, as a sleep aid, or just to relax from pain and stress. It was even used as a love passion. Marijuana mixed with other herbs and drugs was take by a newly married couple on their first night. In the fifteenth century the tribes that lived at the same time that the Maya's were in power. These tribes depended survival totally off of the land and their environment. The people used the hemp plant to make rope, clothes, and many other uses. Marijuana leaves have been found inside of Amber that was dated as to be over one million years old. Marijuana seeds were found in a Egyptian burial tomb that was ten thousand years old. As human beings advance with more knowledge and learn better was of treating illnesses, they put aside the knowledge of the past and don't utilize it and it is forgotten. In ancient times, humans suffer from the same if not more illnesses as people today. The major difference is today there are much more medicines available to treat illnesses, then in the past. It is true that modern medicines triumph over herbal medicines but herbal medicines still have their uses.

MARIJUANA TAX

The underground marijuana market indicates that the annual American marijuana trade is estimated close to $120 billion dollars. It is estimated that it cost Federal and State governments close to 25 billion dollars in fighting the war on drugs and if the change to make marijuana legal then a large amount of that money could be used for more important matters. Of cause these estimations are not accurate due to the fact that all illegal drugs are lump together like cocaine, heroin, crack, illegal pills. It is obvious these days to most people that marijuana doesn't fall in the category of these other more harmful drugs. The potential taxable money derived from taxing marijuana is estimated at about 20 billion dollars a year. But these are just estimates and unknown, and could even be much more than 20 billion dollars annually.

First the States and Federal government would legalize medical marijuana and then tax it. One the government realizes that a great amount of tax revenue can be derived, that's the first step and then the second step would be to legalize marijuana for medical use. It is obvious and a fact that marijuana is the most popular drug in America and about 75% of other countries in the world. If marijuana was legalized, law enforcement would be able to concentrate on other crimes and utilize their time in fighting major crime. It would put marijuana drug dealers out of business and create many new jobs that are legal. The States and Federal government would reap the benefits from regulating and taxing the sales of marijuana.

One California retail marijuana club has started increase revenue that totals a half million dollars in one year and 80,000. dollars a year in sales taxes to the State. The Federal Government still does not acknowledge the legitimate commerce that could be gotten from the taxing of marijuana. While legalization, decriminalization and the medical use of marijuana continue to be debated by law makers and policy analysts are thinking about the economic benefits of regulating and taxing marijuana. It is a no brainer to legalize marijuana for medical use but the problem lies with none medical use. As time is ticking away, even now as you read this, things are changing. Every year there are a few States that petition for the legalization and use of marijuana for medical use. And every year these States get a little closer to getting the bill past. And every year the bill is almost past but is not. There will come a time when the when the medical marijuana bill will be pasted and this will be a topic of the past. It seems to me that the v taxation and regulation of medical marijuana is a win, win situation to increase the tax revenue with a new taxable item. Maybe in a few more years when marijuana is made legal for medical use instead of law enforcement spraying the herbicide parquet to kill marijuana crops, they will be spraying plant food to grow more plants and bigger.

THE STREET CHEMIST

Street Chemist: Interview with a Street Chemist. A Street Chemist is just another name for street drug dealer. The drug dealer that was interviewed was far from a street dealer but well established and organized, has exclusive customers of all types and categories. Let's call him Joe. Joe has been selling marijuana for many years exclusively. He only deals with different types of marijuana with different potencies. Joe customer's always know how to contact him for a purchase. Joe has been dealing with the same customer's for years and never have a problem because the deals and done low key. Joe's customer's range from the average person to Lawyer's, stock brokers, AIDS patients, depression patient, cancer patients, arthritis patients, business men, people with stress, people that want to feel better than they are and many others. Joe said that his customer's that have medical illnesses are very dependable and have a medical need that helps their particular medical illness. Joe said he always makes sure that he has marijuana for his customer's that have medical illnesses so they won't be without their medication. Joe is helping these people with medical illnesses so they can deal with the illness. Joe never sold marijuana on the street but never the less he's consider what's called a Street Chemist. Joe and his customers all travel and communicate in the quiet underground world of meeting of the minds which is mutual. That gave birth to a long relationship between each other as well as trust. Joe only did businesses with the people he knows and no one else.

PAST MARIJUANA USE

Once upon a time marijuana was a legal drug before 1937 in the United States. It has been proven that marijuana is the second most popular drug in the world. The first is alcohol. Marijuana is one of the Earths oldest medicines. Ancient Chinese herbalist used it for many illnesses. Marijuana can grow almost any place in the world. The earliest record of its use was in ancient China and India and from there branched out to other places over the world. In 1804 Napoleon Bonaparte's army is introduce to marijuana which is smoked rather than drank like alcohol. The army proffered the marijuana because of no hang over after effects. Marijuana was used as an extract in medicines, put into chocolate candies to ease stomach pains, ease fevers, or any aches at all. Marijuana was used in the paten industry mixed in with home remedies and patent medicines. In 1876 the sultan of Turkey gave a gift to the United States, a large amount of marijuana to celebrate the 100th anniversary of The Declaration of Independence. It was like the World Fair of that time period. At the Turkish pavilion the visitors would be introduced to smoking marijuana and it was excepted from then on. The smoking parlors open up all over the country. There were salons, bars, and smoking parlors at that time. At the smoking parlors, one could smoke marijuana or eat candies mixed with marijuana. Back in those days marijuana was sold like cigarettes, soda candy, and anything else. Then came the probation of alcohol had made marijuana the number one legal drug in the country and yet alcohol still ranks number one in the country as most preferred Marijuana was cheap and very popular. Marijuana would be banned, State by State for one false reason or another. In 1937 the United States past a law banning marijuana. After the banning of marijuana, it went underground for many years but was still used. Even though there were more habit forming and dangerous legal drugs still being sold on the market In the 1960's the marijuana law was canceled. During the 1970's during the baby boomer era, marijuana was the most preferred drug of the 1970's. It came from the earth and was all natural. It's not habit forming with and up feeling. And no over dosing with it. In the late 1960's a lot of young people were over dosing on many different types of drugs during that time period. In 1970 the Controlled Substance Act, was a ban on any type of drug use. So marijuana goes underground once again. Medical marijuana has gained acceptance in the 1990's. 1970 the federal law band marijuana on the ground that it had no medical benefits, but today marijuana is used legally for medical benefits in 11 of the United States. Maybe someday in the 21 century. It can only happen with changing times.

MARIJUANA: A MILD SEDATIVE

Marijuana is said to be a mild hallucinogen but it's effects are more like a mild sedative that depends on the quality and dosage of the marijuana. Some people have stated that feel relaxed and a pleasant feelings of a type of mild euphoria. Marijuana does not lead to physiological dependence, however can lead to psychological dependence. Mentally the person experiences a strong need for marijuana when feeling tense and anxious.

Posttraumatic stress disorder and the trauma of military combat can leave a survivor of military combat in a traumatic state for months and even years after the combat event. Many people surviving the turmoil of war can experience psychological problems following the conflict. These people were suffering from the fear of the ever present threat of death or mutilation, and severe psychological shocks. There are several types of war trauma and reactions to combat. A few terms that are used, combat fatigue, shell shock, war neuroses. Survivors of combat cannot help but be effected after or during a life threatening ordeal. Posttraumatic stress disorder or combat related stress can manifest itself at any time after the combat event. That means that a person in or during or after and even prior to the combat event. With whatever wars are going on right now there will be soldiers with combat stress disorder as it was in the past wars. Depression, irritability, fatigue and difficulty concentrating are some of the symptoms of this disorder. Some people with this disorder will take marijuana as a medication for their problem as well as other medications. Some soldiers that have performed well under intensive combat situations have experienced posttraumatic stress after they have returned home. The trauma of being a prisoner of war is also a life changing experience to a person. Those who survived the ordeal often sustained residual psychological damage with a lowered tolerance to stress of any kind. Reentry into society is difficult for former survivors of a war prison Outside of psychological scars for the rest of their lives and emotional scars are so profound and present. The trauma of being held hostage can be a horrifying ordeal that can leave a person with intense symptoms of anxiety and distress. A large number of people with these disorders will take marijuana to relax themselves from stressful episodes.

THC ACTIVATES RECEPTORS

THC- activates previously unknown receptors in the brain, that affects the mine in different ways. The THC acts like a combination that can open a safe or the exact key that can only open that particular door lock. These receptors in the brain are found in the Hippocampus, which affects memory, and in the Cerebellum which affects movement, and in the Frontal Cortex which affects Thinking. The receptors reacts to the chemicals transmitted in the brain. The receptors communicates with the chemicals that the body makes, but with THC receptors that have never been activated, become activated and function for the first time. This is a new breakthrough in science, that could lead to other breakthroughs for the use of medical marijuana. Scientist are doing testing on THC and how it affects the memory. They want to know if THC can be utilized in cases where people may need to forget certain memories that are detrimental to them. For example in cases where people need to forget a traumatic memory or a type of mental trauma. Another example would be a war time veteran reliving horrible combat memories that will affect him or her the rest of his or her life. The veteran will have the same repetitious nightmares. Another example would be, in certain cases of rape that leave a person mentally traumatized and are tortured and anguish with memories of the attack. Most people take memory for granted and don't give in a second thought. Most people think that it is very important to have a good memory, which is true. But it is just as important to forget none important things. For example, a none important memory like the people that you pass when your walking down a street. You don't want to remember them so your mind uses selective dispatching of none important memories. Parts of the brain act like a tape recorder, that records and stores memories or can erase or delete memories. Scientists are studying the effects of THC to hopefully be able to target and eliminate nightmares from the memory bank in the brain. These are some new studies in this aspect of using medical marijuana in regards to the forgetting process of the mined. These receptors are only activated by THC . Scientist are testing other plants to see if and what receptors may be active that are dormant until they are activated by the plant. I sure there are other unknown and known plants that may be the key to open a different combination to the resistor's lock.

Herbal Medicines Date Back

Human beings have utilized herbal medicines since the beginning of mankind and will continue to use herbal medicines for as long as the Earth yields it. In the 15th and 16th century in Africa there were many tribes like Nudies, Musonis, Unganase, Zulu, Owabie, ext., these tribes all had witch doctors, elder healers whose job was to help the physical and mental and spiritual needs of the people. They would utilize all of nature's bounty in their effects to help there people. They would use all types of combinations of herbs for different treatments of illnesses including marijuana. Herbal medicine combinations have been past down from generation to generation for thousands of years. Even before man learned how to forge metal there were herbal healers taking care of the needs of their people. It was found that in and ancient burial site said to be thousands of years old Archeologist found that marijuana seeds that had petrified. Suggesting that marijuana was used in conjunction with a burial ceremony or ritual. Marijuana was also used for spiritual purposes as well as medical purposes. 500 years ago there were herbal healers in the 14th century Europe one of which was Michel Nostradamus who was not only known for his predictions but for his medical knowledge in healing others. During this time period the people were affected with wide spread contagious disease associated with a high death rate. The disease was called the Black Plague and epidemic disease with high mortality that swept Europe during the 14th century. As a young man Nostradamus would help treat people with this fatal disease with medicines, herbs of all kinds, and clean practices.

Nostradamus experimented with different herbs from 1521 to 1529. During this time period there were no laws pertaining to the use of any of the herbal medicines Back at that time all herbal healers used marijuana at one time or another to treat numerous types of illnesses, mental and physical. In changing times modern man will admit to or realize the medical benefits of medical marijuana as was realized in man's past.

Testing Different Pain Medications

It's funny how these days some modern doctors are experimenting with all types of pain medications and disease fighting medicines such as Bee Sting Venom, Snake Venom of all types of Snakes. Blow Fish Venom, Scorpion Venom, Frog Venom from all types of Frogs and many other types of animals and plants including marijuana. These experiments are going on every day. With changing times and more study on these new investigations and innovated ideas in experiments on these venoms and plants. Very little experimentation is being done on medical marijuana and it's medical benefits. In many other counties they have experimentation of marijuana and it's benefits. Some of these counties have legalized medical marijuana prescribed for pain relief and for numerous different types of illnesses. With changing times this country will catch up with other counties to utilize medical marijuana benefits for people with illnesses of all types. As we enter into the future the legalization of medical marijuana will come to pass and will be seen as long overdue and after a short while medical marijuana will be used in the same fashion as many other illness treatments. As time moves on after the legalization of medical marijuana for the treatment of medical illnesses. This issue will become a thing of the past.

17 LEGAL MEDICAL MARIJUANA STATES:

Alaska, Arizona, California, Colorado, Connecticut, DC, Delaware, Hawaii, Maine, Michigan, Montana, Nevada, New Jersey, New Mexico, Oregon, Rhode Island, Vermont, Washington.

There are 6 more States that are about to vote on the legalization of medical marijuana use for patients with medical illnesses. Each State has similar legalization of medical marijuana with a few differences. Some States will have these as approved medical conditions: Cancer, glaucoma, or positive status for HIV/AIDS when the condition or disease results in symptoms that seriously and adversely affect the patient's health status. Cachexia or wasting syndrome, severe chronic pain that is persistent pain of severe intensity that significantly interferes with daily activities as documented by the patient's treating physician. Intractable nausea or vomiting.

Epilepsy or intractable seizure disorder. Multiple sclerosis, Crohn's disease, painful peripheral neuropathy. A central nervous system disorder resulting in chronic, painful spasticity or muscle spasms. Anorexia/Cachexia, hepatitis C infection, damage to the nervous tissue of the spinal cord with intractable spasticity, Alzheimer's disease, and many other illnesses and medical conditions or its treatment approved by the state Department of Health. The legalization does not cover all the illnesses that medical marijuana can be taken for, but it's a start.

Possession Amounts of Medicinal Marijuana

Each state has its own rules and regulations pertaining to the possession and cultivation of medical marijuana. For example, in the District of Columbia the maximum amount of medical marijuana that any qualifying patient or caregiver may possess at any time is two ounces of dried medical marijuana. The Mayor may increase the quantity of dried medical marijuana that may be possessed up to four ounces. And shall decried limits on medical marijuana of a form other than dried.

In the state of **Maine** patients (or their primary caregivers) may legally possess no more than one and one-quarter (1.25) ounces of usable marijuana, and may cultivate no more than six marijuana plants. Of which no more than three may be mature. Those patients who possess greater amounts of marijuana than the allowed by law are afforded a "simple defense" to a charge of marijuana possession.

In **Rhode Island** possession or cultivation limits the amount of marijuana that can be possessed and grown to up to 12 marijuana plants or 2.5 ounces of cultivated marijuana. Primary caregivers may not possess an amount of marijuana in excess of 24 marijuana plants and five ounces of usable marijuana for qualifying patients to whom he or she is connected through the Department's registration process. In 2009 the creation of compassion centers, which may acquire, possess, cultivate, manufacture, deliver, transfer, transport, supply, or dispense marijuana, or related supplies and educational materials, to registered qualifying patients.

In **Oregon** possession or cultivation a registry identification cardholder or the designated primary caregiver of the cardholder may possess up to six mature marijuana plants and 24 ounces of usable marijuana. And may possess combined total of up to 18 marijuana seedlings.

In **New Mexico** patients have the right to possess up to six ounces of usable cannabis, four mature plants and 12 seedlings. Usable cannabis is defined as dried leaves and flowers, it does not include seeds, stalks or roots. A primary caregiver may provide services to a maximum of four qualified patients under the medical cannabis program.

Alaska patients have the right to possess up to no more than one ounce of medical marijuana. Three mature marijuana plants and three immature marijuana plants. Arizona patients may possess up to one ounce of medical marijuana, six marijuana plants. Half of which should be mature and the other half should be immature.

California patients may have 8 ounces, six mature plants or 12 immature marijuana plants.   Colorado patients have the right to possess 2 ounces of medical marijuana, six marijuana plants, with three or more not mature.

Delaware patients may possess no more than six ounces, and three mature marijuana plants.   Hawaii patients may possess one ounce of medical marijuana, three mature marijuana plants and four immature marijuana plants.

Vermont patients may possess two ounces of medical marijuana, two mature marijuana plants and 7 immature marijuana plants.

Of cause the Federal Government still has the law on the books that medical marijuana is unlawful in these states. So patients are still being prosecuted in these states by the Federal Government, even when medical marijuana is legal by state laws. Does that make sense?

WORDS FOR THOURGHT   world, lithe, extemporaneous, shines, battles, atonement, pathology, lives, bata, audio, fusion, cleaners, suns, moon, clue, mini, dioxin, endmost, propensity, rear, unabled, clone, topically, mars, verins, young, antacid, allure, ablaze, chorusing, luster, manx, nee, wanting, attac, saving, affection, erasing, off, years, alter, tides, seamans, isolate, echo, lavish, slow, trilogy, shine, inactivate, eat, clock, cardiology, olivine, surpasses, tv, global, incoherent, try, adduced, chiefs, merits, vacancies, nerves, holes, verge, sweet, talent, nightmare, formula, if, time, fourth, artificial, psychology, linking, conciliations, vindication, perfectly, ice, mind, reaction, incalculable, anthropoid, decentralize, preservation, design, prerequisite, voyage, timeless, ever, accomplishment, sunshine, pendulum, soul, oscilate, ambiguous, theology, accumulated, philosophic, subduction, genesis, zygote, abomination, crystal, computer, infinity, typhoon, fire, clowd, bobble, transultrasonic, ra,.

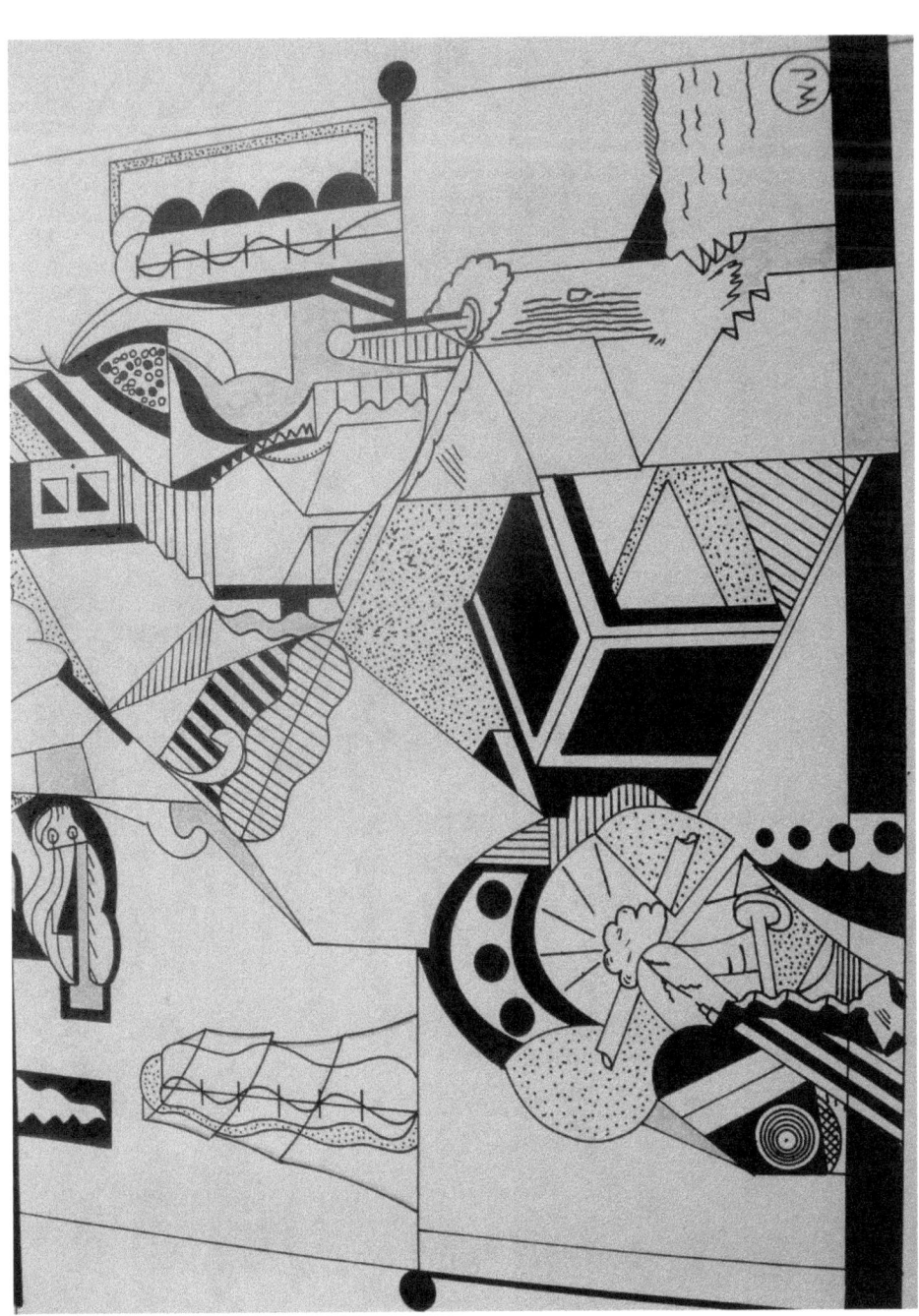

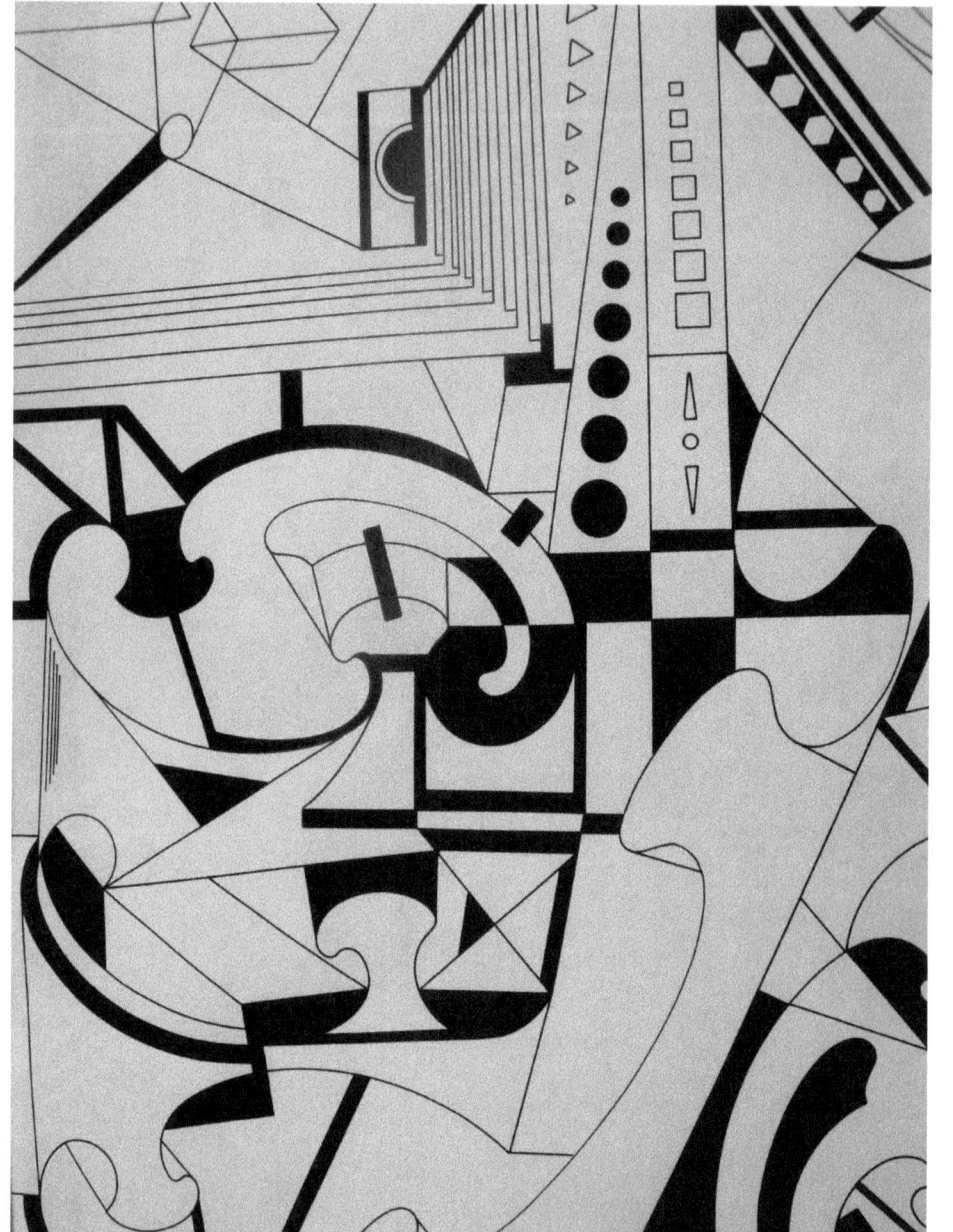

II   Health: Conditions and Diseases

<u>CANCER</u>

KAPOSI'S SARCOMA

Kaposi's Sarcoma is a cancerous tumor of the connective tissue associated opportunistic infections and the immune suppression associated with AIDS. Leukemia in adults has four different forms. Medical marijuana is taken as a appetite inducer for weight loss and anorexia. Herpes Zoster otherwise known as Shingles which is theorized that varicella zoster virus lies dormant in the dorsal root ganglia and is reactivated by and acute illness or emotional stress, trauma, systemic disease like Hodgkin disease. Some people over 50 years old and people who are HIV positive are more likely to develop the disease. Medical marijuana is taken as a relaxer medication.

Testimonials - Breast Cancer

Joan B. suffers from BREAST CANCER

Joan B., a 40 year old widow of two years. Her husband had left her well off so she did not have to work. She began to travel around the world. After six years Joan was diagnose with breast cancer nonmalignant. She had to have a subcutaneous mastectomy. This was very hard for her to deal with mentally but she went ahead and had a Lumpectomy. It was found that the tumors found were not malignant. Chemotherapy and radiation treatment and Joan began to recoup her energy. Joan was still feeling down and thinking to herself that she was less than the woman she was before. She would use the support bra and over compensate with makeup but this did not change her low mood. She decided to go on a trip to Jamaica in the Islands to rest up. While in Jamaica at a beach party she tried marijuana an found that she felt better and more upbeat and a increase in her appetite. After her trip coming back home she began to regress back to a low mood. In the state where she lives there were no legalization of medical marijuana so she perches it through a friend and began growing marijuana in her fruit and vegetable garden.

She began to gain more self-esteem and thinking in a more optimistic way. She soon became a woman's consoler pert time to consol women that are about to go through a lumpectomy or mastectomy and how to deal with it after. She would not tell the women about the marijuana in her garden but she did tell them about all the other treatments that are available.

Jackie R. suffers from BREAST CANCER

Jackie R. is a 37 year old computer programmer that's had her breast removed because of cancer. The doctor's believe they got all the cancer and Jackie would have to be monitored for any recurrence. Having gone through this physical and mental ordeal she needed a very light type of medication. She did not wish to take any antidepressant pills or alcohol medication. She began to take marijuana as a gentle medication without after affects such as hang over or stomach cramps. Having a house in the country she would constantly work on the property as well as her garden in which marijuana was also cultivated. Jackie's mastectomy had left her with fear and anxiety as well as lack of mobility of her arm and shoulder. In Jackie's case the cancer did not spread to any other areas and yet the fear is still there. Jackie would go to mental therapy as well as physical therapy as she would say to get her life back together again. She would have bouts of depression that she would have to deal with and over come. She even thought about having breast implants to maybe satisfies the void she felt. Jackie would soon get a man that loves her as she is and that she falls in love with.

Testimonials - Other Cancers

Stacy S suffers from CANCER

Stacy S. is suffering from stress from having cancer at the age of 52 years old. She has been living with cancer for some time and is dealing with it the best she can. She had found out that the cancer was none malignant which gave her a little relief. She still has stress and fear of cancer. The stress affects the (ANS) autonomic nervous system. This controls regulating, a wide variety of functions like heartbeat, blood pressure, glands, muscles, internal organs, respiration, and gastric-acid-production. Stacy has nausea at times. She has physiological reactions to stress that is detrimental to her body. She also recently went throw a divorce which added to her stress. She has feelings of being obsolete, over the hill, not a young women anymore and afraid of not being attractive to men any more. These things are all incorrect, and all in her mind which could be changed. Stacy went to talk therapy sessions were she met a women named Liz that would turn into a good friend. The two women spent a lot of time together helping each other. Liz has cancer to and her cancer is in remission. The two women would go shopping and hang out together some times. One day Liz noticed that Stacy wasn't looking well and asked her, how is she feeling? Stacy said that she had nausea from stress as well as menstrual cramps. Liz gave Stacy some marijuana in some herbal tea mix to help with the stress and nausea and menstrual cramps. Stacy's stress soon disappeared as well as the nausea. These are some other herbs that are taken for these ailments. Artemisia vulgaris, Camptotheca acuminate, Catharanthus roseus, may apple, roseroot, arctic root, ginkgo biloba, Podophyllum peltatum, Taxus baccata, T. brevifolia,.

Communication, Endocrine and Mental Disorders

ANXIETY DISORDER

Anxiety Disorder is described as an exaggerated feeling or sensation of doom, dread, or uneasiness. Overwhelming anxiety can result in generalized anxiety disorder uncontrollable unreasonable worry. People suffering from generalized anxiety disorder live in a constant state of tension, worry, and irritability, tense, on edge feeling, difficulty sleeping, and sore muscles. Medical Marijuana helps with this disorder in many ways. It helps by relaxing the tension, as well as the ability to sleep and also helps eliminate worry and irritability.

Everyone has had anxious moments in their life weather good moments or bad moments. It is a normal reaction to have an anxiety attack over a problem but it is not

26

consider normal to have anxiety neurosis. Anxiety neurosis is a functional disease which symptoms are somatic thoughts of fear that era manifested out of proportion to extreme fear and frustration out of proportion can lead to anxiety state. A person with this disease can experience symptomatic complains like heart pain, head aces, nerves cold, hot, sweaty an other symptoms. This is not a physical disease or organic disease but a mental disorder which is treatable. Another form of this disorder is anxious agitated depression which symptoms are lack of sleep, depression, agitation, worry, delusions, panic. There have been reports indicating that people are taking medical marijuana to treat these illnesses. As well as other herbal medicines like American Ginseng, Asian Ginseng, Ashwagandha, Gotu Kava, St. Johns Wort, and many others.

Testimonials - Anxiety

Sandy S. suffers from ANXIETY NEUROSIS

Sandy S. a 32 year old female suffers from anxiety neurosis (a troubled feeling or experiencing a sense of dread or fear of the future or distress over a real or imagined threat to one's mental or physical well being). Her anxiety neurosis is manifested when fear of not being able to solve a problem. She complains of heart pain, sweating, pressure about the head. She has a functional disease in which the somatic evidences of fear are amplified out of proportion to the apparent extremes. The real significance is a feeling of inadequacy in dealing with some situations. Sandy had been taking therapy, counseling and medications for several years as well as marijuana as one of the medications to help her maintain normal daily life. Sandy stated that when she had taken the marijuana it calmed her down to a level where her mind did not rush into imaginary tangents. She began practicing mental exercises which were to concentrate thinking of happy and positive thoughts. In doing this it eliminates a lot of fear and negative thoughts.

The marijuana as a relaxing affect as well as an upbeat felling. Sandy's boyfriend Warren would help her when he could but he did not fully understand Sandy's problem's. Never the less he would be supportive to her. They would see each other on the weekends

27

or when their schedules permitted. Warren is a traveling salesman that would travel constantly. When in town Warren would go to see Sandy as well as call her on the phone when not in town. Their relationship has been on and off for years but Warren still comes back. Warren does not take marijuana but he understands why Sandy takes it for her illness. He noticed that Sandy was less moody and more upbeat about things.

Calvin R. suffers from ANXIETY ATTACKS

Calvin R. suffers from anxiety attacks for most of his life. Calvin is 27 years old working as a sales person in a large Mall. He also would have panic attacks that would cause him to have over whelming feelings of worry or fear. He would complain of muscle cramps, heart beating fast, when there was no physical cause. Calvin would go from doctor to doctor and get the same response that was the same. He went for mental counseling and was diagnosed with anxiety. He was having panic attacks sometimes frequently that would affect the way he was thinking and what ever thought conclusions he came to, which most of the time was incorrect. Some people that have panic attacks in this state are not thinking and reasoning in the right frame of mind. Calvin started taking antidepressant medications which helps with anxiety attacks. The medications began to decrease the amounts of anxiety attacks that Calvin was experiencing. He was more relaxed under the antidepressant medications but he would complain about physically feeling drugged up and groggy. Calvin discontinued he medication that was making him groggy and continued taking those medications that wasn't. He also was taking marijuana to relax him and his mind. Calvin would also take the herb Elderberry for his nervous condition and Gotu Kola herb that improves mental support for anxiety and St. John's Wort herb.

Depression

DEPRESSION

There are many types of depression which are basically the same only in different degrees. There is mild depression and heavy depression and all the levels in between. Tens of thousands of people will take medical marijuana for their form of depression. Many of these people were prescribed drugs that they said made them groggy and over medicated to a point that they could not cope with daily life. They chose to stop the prescribed drugs and take medical marijuana instead.

Depression turns into a down feeling and low mental state of mind which can affect ones physical state as well. There are a large number of people with decreased mental and physical energy. We live in a cause and effect world and it is the same with a depression illness. Having a depression illness causes physical problems as well like loss of weight due to loss of appetite. Difficulty falling asleep or sleeping too much. Some depressed people will over eat due to the illness and gain too much body weight. The mental condition is definitely lined to the physical condition. Premenstrual syndrome (PMS) in some women have an irritability abdominal pain as well as full blown depressive illness, have a sense of hopelessness, decreased energy and impaired concentration. There are a few women whose cycle mood disorder becomes linked to the menstrual cycle. These women usually have a rather abrupt onset of symptoms of depression or mania. They will take medical marijuana as a relaxer and to increase appetite and as a pick me up feeling.

Agitated Depression

AGITATED DEPRESSION

Agitated depression is a psychiatric depression that symptoms are restlessness, feelings of guilt, depressed, phobias, obsessions and ideas of being persecuted. This is very similar to manic depressive patients. Meningitis virus causes loss of appetite which treated with marijuana put in tea so that the patient does not get a head ace. To beat this virus the patient must eat food in order to maintain strength. There are many types of depression which are basically the same only in different degrees. There is mild depression and heavy depression and all the levels in between. Tens of thousands of people will take marijuana for their form of depression. Many of these people were prescribed drugs hat they said made them groggy and over medicated to a point that they could not cope with daily life.

They chose to stop the prescribed drugs and take marijuana instead. Depression turns into a down feeling and low mental state of mind which can affect ones physical state as well. There's a large number of people with decreased mental and physical energy. We live in a cause and effect world and it is the same with a depression illness. Having a depression illness causes physical problems as well as loss of weight due to loss of appetite. Difficulty falling asleep or sleeping too much. Some depressed people will over eating due to the illness and gain too much body weight. The mental condition is definitely linked to the physical condition. Premenstrual syndrome (PMS) in some women irritability abdominal pain and full blown depressive illness, a sense of hopelessness, decreased energy and impaired concentration. There are a few women whose cycle mood disorder becomes linked to the menstrual cycle. These women usually have a rather abrupt onset of symptoms of depression or mania. They will take marijuana as a relaxer and to increase appetite and as a pick me up feeling. People suffering from mania feel that their thoughts are racing through their mind. They have constant changes in mood, inflated self images, take ill-advised chances, buying sprees, reckless driving are all common. Suffering from mania depressive illness one alternate between depression and mania which is its opposite. A person having an episode of depression can be followed immediately by an episode of mania or the other way around. Major depression and mania depressive illness are common and can strike any one. About 10 percent of Americans will experience an episode of major depression at some time during their lives. This mood disorder causes to much energy accompanied by extreme happiness or irritability. A person suffering from mania may develop anger beyond irritability, like to talk excessively sometimes jumping haphazardly from idea to idea. They may wake up refreshed. Many of these people will take marijuana to aid in relaxing illness and calming their mind.

Lora I suffers from DEPRESSION

Lora I. is a 37 year old mother of two children that is suffering from depression after the separation from her husband. The children are a boy 8 years old and a girl 11 years. The reason why Lora and her husband, Brad are separated is infidelity on Brad's part. Brad has had several affairs with other women and was asked by Lora to leave the house. So Brad moved out and rented a small apartment. They have been separated for several months and this caused Linda to go into a deep depression. At first Linda had a lot of anger over Brad's affairs with other women and then she started to think that the separation was her fault. She thought maybe it was something that she did wrong or maybe she was not being a good wife. Or maybe she let the fire out of their marriage. Or maybe because she had put on more body weight over the years and was not attractive to him anymore. Or some ting else that she did wring. Thinking the way she is thinking, as if she did the wrong thing in their marriage instead of Brad. She began to think that she would try to change herself to more of what Brad wants in a woman. She still loved Brad and wanted to save the marriage. So she picked a certain day to go get her hair done and make up done and put on a dress that Brad liked to see on her. She decided to drop by Brad's apartment and surprise him with her visit. She drove over to his apartment right after it got dark that evening. When she got to the apartment she knocked on the door and the door opened. Standing there was a woman with nothing on but Brad's shirt. The women asked Lora, may I help you? Lora looked at the women with shock, and said no, no I must have the wrong apartment. And just then Lora herd Brad's voice say, who is it honey? Lora said I'm sorry I'm at the wrong apartment and she quickly turned and went back to her car. Lora was devastated, and started crying as she sat in her car for a good ten minutes before driving home. Lora did not know that Brad was living in the apartment with another woman. That's when Lora's depression really took hold. Lora felt sad and was broken hearted once again by Brad. Soon after that Lora was sleeping late in the morning where as the children would wake her up in the morning before going to school. The children noticed the fast change in their mother and it began to affect them. The children were starting to worry about their mother. After all the children were affected by their parent's separation as well.

Lora would not seem to care about herself and started to let herself go. She would look at TV all day and not have an interest in normal activities. At times she would be irritable and take it out on the children and then she would apologize to the children and said, I'm sorry, mommy don't feel well. The depressed mood and feeling of sadness had taken hold. The children decided to call their aunt Linda to come out to visit them. Once Linda got to the house which was a mess, she knew something was wrong. When she saw Lora, Linda said, you look terrible sis. What happened to you? Lora said, I've not been feeling well these days. Linda knew right away the signs of depression in her sister. Linda began to take charge and said I'm going to help you sis. Let's talk some girl talk while we clean this house up. The next few hours the two women talked and by then Linda knew what the story was. It took a little time for Linda to convince Lora to go with her to get professional help. By this time Lora's mental condition was in the depth of depression, low self-esteem, hopelessness, worthlessness, and feelings of guilt. Linda took Lora to a psychotherapist for counseling. The therapist prescribed some medication and psychotherapy. Even though Lora seemingly fell into a depression over night it will take a lot longer to get out of it. It will take time. It was good that Lora has someone like her sister Linda to help. Some people have no one to help. Linda would come over to her sisters, help out with the children, and make sure that everything was starting to get back to some sort of normalcy. Linda would make sure Lora made it to the counseling sessions and took her medication. The counseling sessions were having a good effect but the medication Lora didn't want to take. Lora told her sister to get her some marijuana. Lora said to her that she needed a much lighter medication than what was prescribed. Lora would take the marijuana instead of the other medication. She either smoked it or mixed it with hot green tea. After sometime had passed Lora was ready to join the world again. She began to feel better about herself and gain back herself esteem. She would continue to take marijuana until her depression had passed. She would stop taking the marijuana because she knew that marijuana is not habit forming like other drugs. Lora would soon be ready to go back to work and do the things that she loved to do. After about two years had passed, Lora and Brad's divorce was final. Lora got her life together again and even found a new man that worships her. Everything was going great for Lora and then one Sunday while Lora and her new man were looking at TV when there was a knock at the door. Lora went to see who was there, and it was Brad. As she looked at him through the peep hole of the door, he didn't do well. She opened the door and Brad said that he had something important to tell her. She said to him what happened to you? You look bad. Brad said that's what I want to talk to you about. Lora took Brad into the kitchen while her new man was watching TV in another room. Brad sat down at the kitchen table and proceeded to tell Lora what was wrong. It had been found that he was HIV positive from one of his sexual exploits and he wanted to get some of his affairs together just in case. Lora told him that she and the children would help all they can. And she also informed him that she has a new life and was happy, and what she and he had in the past was over between them and can never be renewed. More times than not the old saying, (what goes around comes around) is so true.

Mr. Pompeii suffers from MOOD SWINGS AND DEPRESSION

Mr. Pompeii Monclair is 32 years old suffering from Mood Swings and Depression. Pompeii is a Real Estate sales person that works for a top area Real Estate firm. Due to the poor economical situation, in the past two years in that area the Real Estate Market has dropped. This put Pompeii in a bad financial situation and he was forced to seek other employment. Pompeii is the father of a three year old boy. Pompeii is divorced from his wife and pays child support for his son. Paying child support and all the other bills he has are hard to pay when there is no money coming in. Pompeii's life seems to be on a downward spiral. Pompeii got a part time job, working in a fast food place, working nights to help pay his bills. Pompeii would do his 9 to 5 work week at the Real Estate office these days finding apartments for renters and is not showing or selling houses or property due to the recession and no buyers. Every day Pompeii's situation got worse and worse. The presser on Pompeii began to plumb it down more and more in mood swings of depression. His attitude began to change, he had less time to do the thing that he liked to do in the past. In his mind everything happen at once. Separating from his family and living along, working two jobs that are not profitable, living from pay check to pay check. And now the Real Estate office had cut down his full time job down to part time job. Pompeii began to feel like he was on a sinking ship that was going down a little each day and eventually sunk. Pompeii was not ready to give up yet and began to think of all his options. He had some ideas but was not sure on what to do. His relationship with his e-wife was over and he would see his son once a week and sometimes twice a week. He tries to be a good farther to his son and bond with the boy for the short time he is with the boy. He will not admit it but he feels bad about not being with his son more often. As time moved on Pompeii had met a young lady that would come into the fast food place and began to date. Her name was Ashley, Ashley would become Pompeii salvation. Ashley is a 26 year old College student that's studying business. Ashley is a very active young lady always doing something or any other. Ashley has a type of inner beauty of innocence, that's the type of person that would help a homeless person to their feet or stop to help an injured bird on the ground, she has a good heart. She knows that she can't save the world from its ills, but she believes in help if she can. Ashley seems to be the opposite type of personality of Pompeii, but sometimes opposites work out well. Ashley had dated Pompeii for several weeks and saw the signs of depression in Pompeii and made it her mission to help him with it. Ashley notice that Pompeii was having difficulty sleeping and seem to be losing body weight from a lack of appetite. With Pompeii's type of depression, he began to sacrifice himself to maintain his bills and child support for his son. His condition was having a cause and effect situation with him which Ashley felt had to be turned around. Ashley is very outgoing and can be persistent when she has something set in her mind until completion or salved. Whereas Pompeii is quiet, passive, and unsure on what to do about his situation. They are opposites to each other and yet they get along great together. Ashley knew that Pompeii couldn't afford private depression counseling so she arranged through the College for Pompeii to get free counseling at the free Clinic in his area. The visits to the free Clinic began to help him with his sleeping problem but he still was losing body weight because of lack of appetite. Ashley being the dominant one in their relationship set up an eating schedule for Pompeii to gain back his body weight, which was starting to work.

Ashley made sure that Pompeii had all the kinds of foods that he liked to eat. And then she would be like his special coach when it comes time to eat. If she didn't coach him into eating food he wouldn't get hungry for food and not eat. Of cause Ashley had to spread out her day to accommodate all the things that she had to do. Ashley also gave Pompeii marijuana to help his lack of appetite which was working. The marijuana also comb his nerves and help his to think of positive things verses negative things. Ashley was due to graduate from College and had plan to start a new profession out of State. After telling Pompeii of her plans about moving out of State for a new profession. Ashley made a statement to Pompeii to come with her and start a new like together. Pompeii thought for a few seconds and said yes. That a great idea and I happy you asked me to go with you. After a short time Ashley and Pompeii had fell in love. And began to think of the future together. Pompeii continued to take marijuana maybe three times a week when he had a lack of appetite. Whatever Sate Ashley decides to go to Pompeii could take his Real Estate license with him to applied. Pompeii stated to plan as well. Ashley got a job in Virginia so Pompeii began to scout out that area that they were moving to. They moved to Virginia and Ashley was settling into her new job and Pompeii got a job at a local Real Estate office and getting into the flow of working again. Pompeii would still continue to take marijuana when he felt the need to, to induce hunger. Finally Pompeii was court up on the child support for his son and other bills that he had paid off. The depression and worry had left Pompeii, and he feels good about a new future for him and Ashley. As time moved on they both advanced in each of their professions. After a year Ashley had received a promotion and increase in pay. And in the same time Pompeii was doing very well in the Real Estate office. He was showing houses and properties and making the sale. Being a Real Estate sales person he had access to all the good deals on the housing market so he and Ashley decided to buy a house together and did. They agreed to start a family and have children in the future and get married. Pompeii had stopped taking marijuana at this point and had no need for it any more. Being that marijuana is not physically addictive so he was able to just walk away from taking it. Ashley knew at the time when she first introduced marijuana to Pompeii that it was illegal in their State and could be prosecuted by the laws of that State if they had it in their passion. Ashley knows that the State and Federal laws pertaining to medical marijuana need to be up dated and changed to accommodate medical patients that need its help. Ashley knows that time never stands still and is always moving on. So should certain laws pertaining to medical marijuana in these changing times that we live in. She knows that it was against the laws of that State but in her mind she would take the chance of being arrested to help Pompeii with his appetite problem. The State that they relocated to did allow medical marijuana with the proper papers. But the Federal Government laws haven't yet change pertaining to medical marijuana but the laws will change soon and this will be a thing of the past.

Brenda C. suffers from DEPRESSION

My name is Brenda C., I am a 26 year old female suffering from heavy depression and this is my story, my alarm clock went off even though I was in a half awake dream. I was hesitant to acknowledge the beginning of another day that was sure to be just as dreary as the one before and the one to follow. I got out of bed thinking about the odd feeling that had been creeping around inside my mind for the past month or so. I couldn't pinpoint this feeling or what caused it, why it had suddenly appeared out of nowhere. It seemed to be growing day by day, it was like a dark shadow across my mind. This felt different from simply being tired after staying up too late the night before.

I wasn't always this way before the depression came into my life. I was the type of person who liked to play, laugh and sing. I grew up in a close family, with a Mom, Dad, older brother and two Bassett hounds. My memories from early childhood are mostly happy ones, but by the time I was twelve the atmosphere in my family had started to change. I no longer spent much time with my Dad. He worked the night shift and even when he was around, he usually was in a bad mood. Looking back, I realize that he had began to experience his own problems with depression. But at the time, I was simply hurt and confused.

When I was a senior in High School my mom loaded up my brother and me and moved to my parents Midwestern home town. My Dad followed a few months later after our old house sold. It didn't take long before I gained a reputation at my new school for being different. But nothing had prepared me for the heavy clouds of depression that rolled into my life midway through my senior years, such as one morning I felt a crushing sense of hopelessness that was unlike anything I had ever experienced before. I was envious of the way my brother had everything under control. I thought there was no possible way he would ever let a dark cloud settle upon his brain. But once out in the student parking lot it hit me that I had never felt this way before. Lately, all it took was a tiny set back and I would find myself. Choking down a gush of tears. It happened just the afternoon before basketball practice, the coach hollered at me, for no reason, why does that have the power to affect me this way? What's wrong with me? I wondered. As the weeks went by, it became harder and harder to wake up in the morning. My mind felt cloudier with each passing day. When I could I would go to the school art room. I felt safe there it was my greatest source of comfort. On one typical day I was trying to make it through class without getting into any trouble. But as the weeks passed I felt like something had seized control of my mind. I was always so tired but sleep was hard to come by. I had no appetite, my vision seemed to be growing worse, and my brain felt unable to absorb new information.

Meanwhile my hearing seemed to be growing super sensitive, to the point where the sounds of a typical day were often an agony to endure. Somehow, I didn't think these changes were a normal part of puberty. The darkness was spreading inside me like a cancer. I was radiating negativity on the outside as well as the inside. Family and friends had started to notice the change in me. My mom noticed that school was becoming more and more of a challenge. By the end of the spring semester, my grades had slipped, and I had lost a lot of weight. My physical symptoms were worsening, and I was too run down to interact with others. I just wanted to be alone in my misery. Now that summer was a pond us, we were headed to a family reunion at a relative's home in Florida. I had been looking forward to this trip for months. Everyone was so glad to see each other after years of being apart, the house was full of laughter and storytelling and a few of us walked down to the beach to catch the sunset, suddenly, a dark thought came to mind that I shouldn't enjoy this because soon I have to leave and return to your sad existence. I recognized the source of that thought, that dark force that had seized control of my life. At that moment, I understood that it didn't matter where I was or what I was doing because I would carry this dark cloud around. Looking back, I wonder why b it took so to recognize depression.

The summer before college I was glad to be leaving High School. One day, I was taking a nap on the couch, when suddenly I was awakened by the phone ringing it was my friend Lisa on the line. She wanted to know was I still coming to her Birthday party. Instantly, I was struck by a wave of dread and anxiety, but I'm her best friend and what kind of best friend would I be if I missed her Birthday. So I went. The moment I got there it took every ounce of energy just to act normal. I felt like the saddest person in the world. As the night went on and people started to leave, Lisa knew all about my situation with my depression. She waited till everybody left the party so she could have a private conversation with me. She started telling me to try herbal remedies and medical marijuana . She gave me some and showed me how to smoke it. Almost instantly I felt relaxed and calm. I couldn't believe how relieved I felt. My Mom was very worried about me, she could see my symptoms. So as soon as I got home my Mom made a few calls. She realized I needed professional help. She set up an appointment with a mental health professional. The mental health professional recommended a therapist and drug therapy. So now I had hope antidepressants therapy, and medical marijuana. I knew that I was on the road to wellness. Fortunately, Brenda was able to feel happy again with the help of medication and psychotherapy and medical marijuana to treat the depression and the anxiety. In the process she learned a lot about depression and realized how common it was. To share what she had learned with others, she started a campus group for other students in similar situations. Say's Brenda, the problem is people don't talk about depression, so you end up thinking you're crazy. What really helped her was knowing that there were other people out there who had been through the same things and knew what I was feeling.

Lyn R. suffers from DEPRESSION

My name is Lyn R. and I don't know anything about depression until I was hit with it in a big, big way. I had my first major depressive episode in 1990, but at that time, I didn't know what depression was. I didn't know anybody else who had it, so I had no idea what was wrong with me. I thought I was the only person in the universe who felt the way I did. If I had known more about depression from the beginning, I might not have suffered as long and as hard as I did. Now my mission is to get the word out and let people know that having depression is not a taboo. After all, it seems like half the population is on antidepressants! My illness began after a long- term committed relationship ended abruptly. My companion and I owned a house together, and we were raising a child. I was very involved in my community and I was also a singer in a very popular band. All of a sudden it was all gone. After my companion told me that they wanted to live separately, I went emotionally downhill in three days. I was in total blackness and despair. I didn't understand what was happening to me. I had never been so depressed before. Breaking up with someone is a common life situation, but I wasn't living in reality. Imagine what it's like to have no control of your brain. It's scary. Something in my brain was broken. But mental illness isn't like a broken leg. You can't just put on a cast and fix it. The week after my relationship ended, I moved from New Jersey to my parents home in Florida. I needed to be taken care of and I needed unconditional love. I thought whatever is happing to me will go away in a week or two. But it didn't. I went through torment for almost a year. At first I couldn't eat, I couldn't sleep. I lost about forty pounds in a few months, and I probably only slept about forty hours in that entire time. Most women like myself that were overweight would be happy to loss forty pounds of body weight, but that wasn't me. The only thing I could manage to do was take a shower in the morning. I think what actually got me in the bathroom was looking in the mirror at my body. I would see myself and think that's not me. I was an emotional roller coaster, and I was suicidal for over a year. I should have been in a psychiatric hospital, I lost my job and, with it, my health insurance. I didn't get adequate help at first. I went to see a therapist who did me a terrible disservice. You would think that a mental health professional would have had the sense to put me on medication. Meanwhile I was spending most of my time curled up in a fetal position sobbing. I couldn't function at all, and I suffered deeply. Three hellish months later, I finally saw a therapist who put me on medication.

I was hesitant about taking drugs, because I didn't know anything about antidepressants. They weren't even a part of my vocabulary back then. I didn't want to take any medication because I thought it might alter my mind. Well my mind was already severely altered. I didn't know that my depression was for more than just grief for my lost relationship. I didn't know I had an illness. I certainly didn't know that I couldn't get over it by myself. I met my current friend three years ago, and I told everything about what I was going through, and that's when I found out About medical marijuana, that I should try it.

I was hesitant at first but I tried it, almost immediately I felt relief. Thanks to my medications, the therapist I was seeing, and my parents. I gradually began to get better. My parents are the reason I'm alive today. They were supportive, they loved me unconditionally and they stuck with me even though they knew there was something terribly wrong with me, and at the time, they felt helpless. What did they see when they looked at me? They saw a person who used to be full of life but was now dead inside. They saw me crying and begging for help for hours on end. There is mental illness in my family. I have a nephew who is manic-depressive, and my uncles wife hasn't been able to really function well for thirty years. So mental illness is not something my parents are unfamiliar with. My parents didn't keep my depression a secret. They had a huge community of friends, and I met them all. I wasn't ashamed that I was sick, and I was very verbal about what was going on with me at times. For the last month or so, it's completely uphill for me.

Later I've been feeling one hundred percent myself thanks to medical marijuana and my medication. When I was depressed, I couldn't deal with the baby because I was so sick. I couldn't do anything for myself. Now that I am OK, since I've been with Ben, I've become more open about my own depression and because of Ben I can actually describe what I'm feeling. In the past it n was just a long silent struggle for me. There is depression in Ben's family, his father has depression and his brother and sister has also struggled with it. His sister has bouts of suicidal thoughts for the last four years. She's seeing a therapist and is doing much better. She's even earned her Master's Degree in social work. Ben comes from a family where you shut up and buck up. Her mom has a lot of issues about what other people think. She is really into how you present yourself to the world. Medical marijuana and medication has helped me tremendously, I was so relieved. I didn't feel like a freak anymore. Finally, I knew that there was nothing to be ashamed of. Recently I've started work again' and I'm able to do accounting and auditing easily. Now I can drink a beer with friends, socialize, do karaoke, and go to parties. But even today my world is small. I'm not particularly optimistic about the good graces of humanity. There are good and bad people out there and if someone chooses to use my illness against me, that's their problem. I don't feel that I have to reveal all that much about my illness to other people. It's part of my life and something I have to deal with on my own. God has sent a lot of people my way who have helped me enormously. I've had good role models in my church who have supported me, and the biggest thing I've learned is compassion for others. If I come across people who want or need help, I'll give it to them. I still have obsessive thoughts, but with medical marijuana I can control them better than ever before. I can block them out by thinking about something else, or by talking to a friend. I recognize my behaviors now for what they are they're petty, they waste time, and they take away from my life. Some people may not have as much will power as I do, but I think it's possible to change your life, to turn things around for yourself, and to get help if things aren't right.

It's not good to languish in your own problems. That's the worst thing you can do. The church gave me a lot of support and support is what you really need when you have a mental illness. You really need someone to understand you. I think that being religious has helped anchor me. My medications and medical marijuana and my doctor have helped a lot, too, and this is wonderful. I've done remarkably well, I've become a different person. The worlds too big to give up on and I never did that. People think that having a mental illness is a shameful thing, and don't respect you if you have one. I didn't think they should look down on it. People should try to be more open minded and more tolerant to those that my need help. I have been in therapy for a long time, and I talk about the whole circle of guilt that I get caught up in. For instance, sleep deprivation is a trigger for my depression. I got out of my way to make sure I get all the sleep I need.

Joan K. suffers from DEPRESSION

My name is Joan K. and this is my story. My recovery from depression wasn't instantaneous, and it wasn't a nice steady incline, either, instead, it was more like a graph with lots of peaks and valleys, but an overall trend that was heading upward. By my sophomore year in high school,. I felt well enough to function as a student and do the things a person my age was supposed to be doing. It wasn't until my junior year that I felt fully recovered. No one would ever wish to have depression, but I did gain some positive insights from my struggle. It may sound like a cliché, but I hadn't realized what I had until I nearly lost it. Now it was as if someone had hit the reset button of my life. I was back at square one again, and this time, I couldn't wait to get started. During my junior year, I joined the cross country track team just for the experience, even though running had never been a talent of mine. I also took part in school plays, traveled to the West Indies as a volunteer, and created some of my most profound artwork. Around town, I was known for the restored car that my dad and I had finally finished. My one of a kind style had morphed into a sense of independence, individuality, and most of all, confidence. I was socializing again. I spent much of my out of school time alone working on art projects. In school focusing had become a bit more difficult because of all the thoughts and ideas flooding my mind. As far as my mood went, some days were harder than others. When I became stressed out from day to day events, I would start feeling down and discouraged. To combat these feeling I would tell myself take it one day at a time. I reminded myself that a single bad day was not a complete reversal of all my progress. The summer before my senior year, I heard about a work shop being held at a college in the north woods of Oklahoma. The work shop was designed to introduce high school students to professionals who worked in various environmental fields. It sounds perfect for me. I would be able to camp in the deep woods, learn about Native Americans, meet botanists, go wolf tracking, tag song birds, and observe bears. Before this workshop, I wasn't sure whether I wanted to go to college. My art business was thriving. I already had mural jobs lined up for the next year, and if I stayed where I was, it looked as if my reputation as an artist might grow rapidly. But the love of nature was another big part of my total self that I felt shouldn't be neglected.

I applied to the workshop, which had limited space, and I was thrilled to be accepted. Around midsummer, I headed to the north woods. I was nervous about being away from familiar surroundings, I had all the standard feelings that come with going somewhere alone for the first time. On top of that, I had added concerns about my mental health and overall stability. I was honest with my mother about those concerns on the car ride to the workshop, but she reminded me of how far I had come and how much strength I had gained. Within the first five minutes of the workshop, I know I had made the right choice. I was so swept up in the experience that I didn't have time to worry about whether or not I would be strong enough to handle it. I felt comfortable in these new physical surroundings, but it was more than that. I found that most of the people around me I saw being a bit weird as a desirable quality. During my senior year, I continued to enjoy myself and embrace my life.

But now that I had seen a small glimpse of what was waiting beyond high school, I had the itch to move on to other things. I sensed that my life was going to take the road less traveled, but I didn't want it any other way. To their credit, my family always supported me in my aspirations. They believed that I would be able to make it on my own as a professional artist. They saw that I wasn't afraid to take risks, and I knew they would be there to support me if one of those risks didn't pay off. Halfway through my senior year, I completed the journal about my experiences with depression. I had worked on this journal throughout my illness, drawing the images in my mind and thinking of my depression as a beast. One day when my uncle was visiting, he saw the journal. His good heart told him that publishing the journal as a book could help others, and his business sense told him it could be successful. He took a copy of my journal around to a number of publishing companies, but it was rejected by all of them. I wasn't discouraged by this, I had never intended for my journal to be published in the first place. It was simply one way I dealt with depression, a channel for expressing my thoughts and feelings as I struggled with the illness and its after math. My uncle still believed passionately in the power of my story, so he decided to self publish my journal as a book and market it himself. As graduation grew near I was juggling several commitments. Aside from school, I was beginning to promote the book, and I was swamped with art commissions. I had worked hard to build a reputation locally as an artist of all trades, doing everything from painting murals in private homes and businesses. My confidence grew day by day even though I still had depression. I didn't feel quite balanced at time. I think it was depression rearing its ugly head again. I took my meds but it didn't help enough. Over time, though I heard a lot of stories that were filled with pain, and I began to let it get me down. I learned a critical lesson, I had to manage my own state of mind and be aware of when I needed a break. Near summers end, my uncle, my mother and I attended a large book convention in Chicago. While at the convention, I met a literary agent who wanted to represent me. She thought a large publishing house might be interested in my book. Even though I should've been happy about this, my depression was weighing me down. The last weeks of summer were spent with a few close friends. We were all a little nervous about starting our brand new adult lives. I felt very anxious and my brain was erupting with questions and concerns. I was afraid of my new environment and I thought my medicine wasn't working, how would I be able to handle daily life on my own. I told my roommate at college how I felt and my mental illness. She told me she has a boyfriend who is Native American and knows about herbs and holistic medicine. He recommended medical marijuana so I smoked it and I thought to myself if I only knew about medical marijuana before things would be different. Within a couple of weeks I was already facing a problem. After being on medication for a few years I had come to take it for granted. I didn't think about it much anymore. I took my meds along with medical marijuana and my moods felt even. I had trouble getting my medication at the pharmacy in a college town, so I went without it for over a week but thanks to medical marijuana I was calm, I could think rational and concentrate on my school work.

My mother and I had been through a lot together and it was an adjustment for both of us getting along without that daily interaction and support. I know my mother was proud to see how independent I had become. As time went on things back home changed even more. My parents got a divorce, and the first couple of years afterward were extremely difficult for my whole family. Midway through my freshman year at college, I received a phone call from the literary agent, I had met the previous summer in Chicago. She informed me that four major publishing companies were bidding on the rights to my book. Eventually a big publishing company did buy the rights to my book, and over the next few months I worked on fine tuning the illustrations and text. The book was released during my sophomore year at college. It was a challenge balancing my new role as an author as well as being a student. But it was also a gift away to salvage something positive and meaningful from the wreckage of my suffering. Today I'm 26 and it has been 12 years since I first found myself in the grips of the beast. Depression is still an unwanted stowaway in my mind, and I know it probably always will be. But with my meds and medical marijuana I work at managing my illness on a daily basis, and although it isn't always, I usually keep the beast at bay. I hope my story will inspire you to find that last bit of strength within yourself. At times, it may be nearly obscured by the darkness, but it's still there. Use your strength to pull the pain out of yourself and into the world, where you can confront it. This tasks tremendous courage, but start feeling better, hold tight to the knowledge of your progress and never forget the strength and courage that brought you there.

Janet G. suffers from Depression

My name is Janet G., when I was a young child, there was a huge boulder three stories below my bedroom window. I always felt that this boulder was meant to be there so that I could kill myself by falling on it. I felt inadequate and sad when I was as young as seven. I knew something was wrong, but I didn't know what it was. My family was dysfunctional. For instance, my brother always did unusual things with me. Sometimes he would dare me to do things that were extremely dangerous and could even be fatal. He once made me run down the street with a garbage bag over my head. My mother didn't get upset or protect me from him. In fact when I was a little girl, my mother sexually abused me. She told me that my vagina was dirty and she used to scrub me so hard that I couldn't urinate for hours and hours. She had a rule that I wasn't allowed to go to the bathroom at school, so for twelve years, I never even saw what a girl's restroom looked like. When I was a bit older, my brother sexually molested me and told me that our parents would kill both of us if I told them about it. Around, my father used to tell me how ugly I was and that no man would even want me. I would try so hard to be thin, that I wouldn't eat anything at all for weeks at a time. My parents didn't care. I was in all honors classes at school. I was under a lot of pressures from my parents to always get straight A's. If I got one problem wrong on a test, my father would tell me how stupid I was for making a mistake. I never felt that I was good enough.

My serious breakdown occurred when I was fifteen years old. I was so depressed that I dropped out of school. And basically slept for three months. My parents told me, I had to get a job to help out. My father found me a job at a restaurant, but it took me over two hours to get there by public transportation. I worked sixty hours or more a week and I was also responsible for cooking meals at home and cleaning the house. My father beat my brother, my mother and me for years. Once, I accidentally broke a teacup that he got in Paris. He beat me with his belt so brutally that later that night I attempted suicide for the first time. My father grabbed me just as I was going out of the third story window. He made me sleep in his bed that night so that he could keep an eye on me. I needed therapeutic intervention, but my family didn't believe in therapy, so I didn't get any help. I saved enough money from working that I was able to afford to go to a Catholic high school although I was only sixteen, I rented a room that was off campus and supported myself by working on weekends. But eventually I moved back home. When I went to college, I eloped with the first boyfriend I had. Fourteen months into our marriage, I asked him to leave because he started beating me and I know where that leads to. He moved out, thinking that I would take him back or that I really needed him. Six months later he began to stalk me. I had to get a restraining order against him, which he violated several times. He went to jail three times, and each time my father and brother would bail him out, thinking that he was right to pursue his wife, to get back together. After I got a divorce I soon got involved with another man who was also abusive. I began to believe that all men are like that or that's the type of man that will accept me.

I married him three years later, he attempted to kill me when our daughter was two years old and I was pregnant with our son. When my son was six months old, I finally went into a battered women's shelter. The shelter staff was neither supportive nor helpful. At one point, the children and I had pneumonia and they would not even help me get me the hospital. I had to do everything on my own. I asked for therapy, but they said they didn't provide therapy for women in the shelter. After two months in the shelter, I was accepted into a transitional living program for battered women and their kids. It was just temporary housing without any real program in place. It was awful. Four months later I received a rent subsidy and I moved again. This was my third move in nine months with two children under three. Everything was falling out from under me. I was completely overwhelmed, and I started to feel very bad about myself. I was all alone with two young children and I had no one to turn to for support. Although I have had depression most of my life, this time it was far more profound. I decided to go to the local mental health clinic. Where I requested therapy for both my daughter and myself. My daughter was only three years old, but she had observed the beatings I had sustained by her father. The mental health clinic couldn't understand why I was so depressed and I couldn't really explain it. I was not leading the life I had intended. I felt hopeless. I couldn't keep up with all the things that I had to do to survive. I began to feel suicidal because I didn't think that my life was ever going to get better.

From the clinic staff, I got to see a therapist. They put me in group therapy. I still wanted to commit suicide. After several sessions one of the people in my group therapy told me I should try marijuana. She told me how much it helped her and she would bring me some to btry. She told me I could smoke it or drink it like in a tea. A few months later, I found a psychiatrist at a different mental health center. She realized that I needed medical medication to stabilize my condition that and the medical marijuana saved my life. People fear mental illness. I've even lost friends because of it. For those of us who have a psychological disability we are, in a sense trapped in an invisible wheel chair. With the help of medical marijuana I've survived an incredible amount. To raise awareness about the struggles of battered women I've created a red heart pin. All the profits go to provide financial aid to battered women and their children.

Given everything that we've been through together, I'm amazed that my children are thriving. Although I'm on state assistance and we live in poverty, I've managed to have the children attend an excellent private school. Even though I'm open with my children about my disability, I've never shared anything about my mental illness with their friends. I was so proud my daughter didn't feel ashamed of me. My kids are such an inspiration to me. Every time I look in their eyes and I see them gleaming, I think this is what I live for, that look in their eyes.

Ruth B. suffers from DEPRESSION

Ruth B. at the age of 32 years old was diagnosed with a medical condition of depression after losing her young child in a house fire. Ruth suffers from a serious medical illness called depression. She began feeling sad and in a depressed mood, loss of interest and friends. Lost weight and appetite for food. She began being treated for depression counseling and medication. After a short period Ruth began to loss body weight and did not like the medication prescribed for her. She said that the medication made her sleepy and out of it, doped up.

She discontinued using the medication and sought alterative medications such as marijuana. Ruth stated that the marijuana has increase her appetite for food as well as picked up her attitude and making her feel more positive about herself. Medical marijuana helps aid as a antidepressant medication. The tragedy of a patient losing a child is very devastating and sometimes it takes many years for the pain to subside. Ruth began to put her life back together again slowly. She began to eat more and put on weight soon after she would go back to work and began to start the long and tedious process of her recovery. Even though Ruth would start to feel that depression was coming on she would take marijuana that relaxed her and make her feel much less depressed. As time went on Ruth would be out of the depression and not need to take marijuana any more.

Christine B. suffers from DEPRESSION

My name is Christine B.,. When I was a little girl, I knew there were things that I experienced that other people didn't. I had a sense of not wanting to be alive, of wanting my life to be over. I can remember lying in a snowdrift one night when I was six, looking up at the stars and wishing that my life would stop, that everything would just stop. I also remember hiding in a closet and wishing I would die. I didn't think about doing anything to actually hurt myself when I was that young but I kept hoping that my life would end. I got very upset when I started to do poorly in school. My father told me that I wasn't allowed to act sad or cry in our home. None of us kids, not even our mom, were allowed to show our emotions at home. When my mother's mother died, my father got mad at her for crying. I can distinctly remember seeing mom in the bathroom with her head in the linen closet and her face buried in the towels, so nobody would hear her cry. Humor was usually okay with my father, but when I began to fail at school, he punished me by not allowing me to laugh in our house anymore. I couldn't express anger or sadness or be openly happy. In order to survive in my family I learned to hide my feelings. I made my first suicide attempt when I was twelve by over dosing on pills. I called a friend to say goodbye, which I now think was my way of asking for help. Her mother contacted my parents. My father asked me to come downstairs and when I did, he hit me. Then I was locked in the bathroom until my parents took me to the hospital to get my stomach pumped. I overheard my parents talking with the doctor in the hospital. He told them I needed to get help. My father said he'd take care of it. My parents took me home and my father told me I should never discuss what I had done with anyone. I wasn't allowed to tell my siblings, I was grounded for a week.. That's when I started to learn how to keep secrets. As soon as I was old enough, I moved far away from home. My parents live in South Carolina and I moved to New Jersey. From a distance, I was able to see more clearly how horrid my childhood had been. I began to feel a lot of rage toward my parents, so I didn't talk to them for the first couple of years after I moved. For years, nobody that there was something wrong with me. My close friends never knew. My colleagues at work never knew. Nobody knew that I spent most of my life wanting to die. I was always joking around and acting very happy and energetic, but in the back of my mind, I had no desire to continue living. I made two more suicide attempts when I was an adult. The first was when I was twenty-one I had gotten married and it was absolutely the biggest mistake of my life.

My husband kept me isolated from everyone who was important to me. I was in so much pain that I tried to kill myself. I saw a c therapist who diagnosed me with depression and prescribed medication. I was able to talk to him about my childhood. I didn't want to go too far into personal stuff. As soon as my crises was over, I quit therapy and stopped taking my medication. I hated its side effects and I didn't want anyone to know that I was taking drugs for a mental illness. I remarried and then divorced my second husband. I was living alone and I became more and more anxious and depressed. I felt like I had to do something drastic. My second suicide attempt occurred on a cold February night when I put a vacuum cleaner hose in my car and attached it to the muffler. I had a bottle of water, my phone, my comforter, my pillow and my dog. I was all tucked in. When I started the car I thought to myself what kind of crazy, selfish woman would kill her dog? I got out of the car to put the dog in the house followed him in and I called a friend because I was in big trouble. This was the first time that I didn't keep my depression a secret. My two closets friends told me about medical marijuana, I tried smoking it and almost right away it picked up my mood and attitude and gave me other thoughts and alternatives that are positive, smoking the marijuana seemed to give me hope. When I would take marijuana for additive pain relief in conjunction with my regular meds. It was like I hit on the right prescription for me. My life has calmed down now, and I feel at peace for the first time. I take my medication religiously along with the marijuana, see my therapist often, and surround myself with people who accept me. I know who and what is important to me. I know that what I can't get from my biological family, I can get from my two closest friends. They meant the word to me, they are true friends and family. It's always been especially hard for me to talk to anyone about my mental illness. I didn't want to look at myself that way. I used to have this picture of mental illness as a dark, gloomy, ugly thing. I didn't want anything to do with that. That's where my two closest friends were very supportive. They helped me look at my illness in a different way. I've come a long way in the last year mostly because of the marijuana and my meds and especially my two friends. I don't like talking to my boyfriend about my mental illness. He's only supportive to the degree that I let him be. I'm working on trying to include him more, but right now I'm focused mainly on getting and staying stabilized. My goals are not only to make more progress in therapy, but also to be more open with my family. I don't think my father will ever change his ways, because in his mind he thinks he's right in what he believes.

Parson J. suffers from ANGER AND DEPRESSION

Parson J. is suffering from depression which leads to anger then leads to rage. Parson is 17 years old and lives in the inner city where there is constant hustle and bustle of city life every day. Every day where he lives there's constant noise from traffic and daily life. Parson has grown up in this environment with all the mentality of have to survive and try to maintain his sanity as well to stay in school and stay out of trouble so as not to destroy his life like so many other inner city young people have. Parson's mother was a single parent that works two jobs to support Parson and a younger sister. Parson is working a part time job as a store clerk near their apartment. So far he has managed to steer clear of bad influences in his environment thanks to a caring school guidance counselor that saw great potential in Parson and became somebody that influence a positive direction in Parson's life. Fortunately Parson managed to control his anger and depression by taking marijuana for the past few years. He's smart enough to know that he could not afford to be arrested for the possession of marijuana. He knows that there is a double standard with the laws when it comes down to weather a person can afford the proper legal representation in the defense and admonishment from the record of a person that has been arrested for passion of marijuana. In other words, whether or not a person that was arrested for passion of marijuana can afford to pay a lawyer to have the charges dropped or having the record wiped clean. Parson knows that he can't afford to pay a lawyer to have this done so he is extra careful when buying marijuana and smoking it. He knows that his option will always be open for what he wants to do in the future. He knows that if he is arrested and has a criminal record most of his option in the future will be limited. For example he knows that if he had a criminal record he couldn't get a government job or a job in law enforcement or many other opportunities would be denied to him. Parson doesn't drink alcohol or take any other drugs, he finds the marijuana helps him maintain his attitude and clams his feelings when he is starting to feel depression coming on or anger. Parson has seen what had happen to others that had gotten a criminal record and what effect it had on their lives. That record basically destroyed their lives and their futures. They had no idea how devastating this was to their futures. Parson has learned from his friends mistakes. His friends thought at that time a simple passion arrest was no big deal, until years later when it comes back up in the future to bite them. Parson as learn that nothing is really always going to be rosy and promising all the time and life is what you make it. He sees most of the double standards that are not correct like how alcohol is a legal drug that society condone and yet they don't want to acknowledge it great dangers and how destructive it is to a person's life. Parson believes that there is something wrong with this society when it really comes to right and wrong, and the economics involved, which controls the outcome. Parson is just bidding his time until he's ready to go out on his own and some day help to make changes in these current laws pertaining to the legalization of marijuana for medical use. Parson was told that his father died from alcohol and he was a good man with a bad alcohol addiction and he would have lived much longer if he didn't have the addition to alcohol. Living in the inner city can force a boy to become a man very fast and have to make the right chose's or wrong ones in their lives.

Gordon S. suffers from DEPRESSION

Gordon S. is a ex policeman that's suffering from depression after losing the use of his legs after being in a car crash. Soon after the crash he was forced into retirement by the police force. He was devastated mentally and began to drink alcohol on a daily basis. His wife was at odds with what to do about his drinking which didn't help their situation. It was very hard for her to try to adapt to have her husband in a wheelchair and not on his feet. When Gordon would drink alcohol his personality would change to a state where he would blame everyone but himself. Trying to deny the fact that he had been drinking alcohol before the car crash, and that it was his own fault that it happen. His wife was over whelmed with the changes in their lives and found it increasingly difficult to deal with. After being in this situation for several month she was a her wits end and needed some kind of help with saving her marriage. She managed to get counseling for herself and for her husband. The counseling was of tremendous help with Gordon's drinking alcohol problem, as well as helping his wife readjust to the new situations that she was confronted with. The circumstances had changed drastically which they both had to adjust to in order to stay together. Both would have to learn how to give and take. Fortunately his wife loves him enough to deal with the new changes. Even though Gordon had admitted to himself that it was his own doing that put himself in this situation, he still couldn't overcome his depression. He had been taking pain medication on a daily basis for his physical discomforts, but he could take any antidepressant medication or not that he couldn't but he refused to. Both are in their mid thirties and have the option to stay with each other or to separate from each other. It probably depends on how much they love each other. Pattie his wife loves him very much and stayed with Gordon through the good times and the bad ones. Pattie work as a school teacher and made sure that whatever personal problems she and Gordon had she would leave them at home. Gordon's insurance covered the cost of having a in house nurse five days a week until Pattie comes home from school to take over. The nurse would inform Pattie on a daily basis on Gordon's physical and mental condition. The nurse always gave a daily report to Pattie which she stated that Gordon was making good progress with his physical exercises but his mental state of depression remained the same. Pattie knows the man her husband was before he lost the use of his legs, and she sees how his mental condition has change. She always has the thoughts that he might do something drastic to himself like taking his service pistol and shooting himself due to such a low mental condition. It began to effect her more and more to a point where she contemplated leaving him for her own peace of mind. She thought to hang in there a little longer before she made any drastic decisions about her marriage. Just so happen, the next day it was the nurse's birthday which she decided to still go to work to take care of Gordon. The nurse constantly tried to pick up Gordon's spirit ever day with no effect. This particular day the nurse talked Gordon into smoke some marijuana to celebrate her birthday to relax him. It did relax him just enough for him to think of other things, and not have self pity for himself. Gordon found out that the marijuana made him feel better and he liked it. He talked the nurse into buying some marijuana for himself and to bring it the next day. The nurse tried to talk him out of it with no effect. The next week the nurse brought him a ounce of marijuana, which he was very grateful to her for getting it for him. After all, Gordon knew that he was asking the nurse to commit a crime.

The nurse was the kind of care giver that believed in really helping others an she knew that she was committing a crime but she believes the marijuana help Gordon's depression. During the course of that week one day when Pattie came home from school, she noticed the smell of marijuana. She went toured where the smell was coming from which was the bathroom. She knocked on the door and Gordon opened it. He was sitting on the toilet bowl smoking a joint. Pattie said, what are you doing? Gordon looked up at her and said, I'm taking medication to make me feel better, then he said, is that ok with you? Pattie just looked at him for two seconds not knowing what to say, and then she closed the door and went to the bed room. Pattie didn't know what to say, whether to chastise her husband or just go along with the program. She decided to wait and see. When Gordon came out of the bathroom he went to the bedroom and began to explain to Pattie that the marijuana was helping his frame of mind and helping with his depression. He was very talkative more so than usual. It had also made Gordon feel more romantic and sexual. After all Gordon lost the use of his legs but all his other parts still worked. Pattie began to think that there are a lot of benefits to marijuana than just helping Gordon's depression. It had changed his outlook on many things for the better in her eyes. She saw that he was less self-centered, more caring, more hopeful, more romantic, and like the man she first married. Even though she knew that marijuana was illegal to use, she saw that it was actually helping her husband and her marriage. She noticed that Gordon was more relax, more optimistic with dealing with the changes in his life, and was not as depressed as he had been in the previous months before he started taking marijuana. He was a little more acceptant of his situation and was trying to make an effort to improve his life. Gordon would have to continue taking his other medication for pain reliever, and the marijuana didn't inhibit or conflict the pain medications. Naturally, Gordon had been a law officer for several years and knows the laws very well. He knows that he's committing a crime in his State and yet he's willing to take the chance that he, himself would not get arrested for marijuana. As time moved on Gordon had to find another way to buy marijuana because the nurse was relocated to a different area. Gordon called up his cousin to see if his cousin had a connection for marijuana and if he would buy it for him. The cousin knew of Gordon's situation and his condition and was happy to help. Gordon's cousin was into a little bit of everything and to smart to get in any big trouble and had been smoking marijuana for recreational use. Gordon had always stayed clear of his cousin because he had been in law enforcement, but now he was not. The cousin was surprised that Gordon would come to him to buy marijuana, but after Gordon explained the circumstances the cousin understood and was happy to do it. After all the cousin would make money on the transaction and get a new customer. Gordon soon began to read book about medical marijuana and became very knowledgeable about it. So much so that he was planning to start a little garden in his back yard in the spring time and grow his own marijuana, with other vegetable products. Gordon would buy a large amount of marijuana that would last him for several months, before having to purchase more.

After the Christmas season Gordon's wife came home early from school one day and he wondered what was up. She had told him the she had to go to the doctor because she wasn't feeling well. And she was told that she was pregnant. Gordon almost jump out of his wheelchair with joy. He said, I'm going to be a farther, I'm going to be a farther. Pattie began to cry for joy herself, she can remember the last time she has seen her husband so happy. Almost immediately they began to make plans for the new addition to their family. Gordon felt he had a new lease on life and began to call marijuana, medical marijuana because for him it was a medication that save his life. He remember the time he thought about ending his life with his service revolver before starting to take marijuana. He always thanks the nurse for introducing him to marijuana, and credits her and medical marijuana for saving his life, and the new life that was coming.

Bob C. suffer from DEPRESSION

Bob C. is suffering from major depression after his son was killed in war. Bob's wife had died from cancer six years ago and his son was killed, just last year. Bob is 55 years old and has lost his will. To live. He has no other family members to count on for support. Bob had been contemplating suicide several different times but never went through with it. Until one day. Bob's fellow employees knew that there was something wrong with him because of the different tragedies in Bob's life. They care for Bob and are very sympathetic about his situation. If Bob took off a day of work they would call him up on the phone to make shore he was alright. His mood worsened and he began drinking alcohol but it didn't help to make things better but worse. When Bob would take off from his job he would always call the job to inform them that he wouldn't be in. If he didn't call them they would call him at home or his cell phone to make shore he was alright. As they feared it happen one day that he did not respond to their calls and they went over to his house to check up on him. Bob had attempted suicide by a over dose of sleeping pills. Fortunately his friend got to him in time to save his life. Bob's in a hospital and is having a mental evaluation which found that he has affective disorder, major depression. He was assigned a mental Doctor that he would have to see once a week in order to keep his job after he was released from the hospital. The Doctor found out that Bob had depressed moods, fatigue, not able to concentrate and self guilt. He blamed himself for the deaths of his family members, as if he could have change anything. Bob feels that he has nothing else to live for, so the Doctor with help from others would convince Bob otherwise. Bob would have to go to talk therapy sessions also. After a short period Bob would complain about the effects of the ant depression drugs that he was taking . One day at one of the talk therapy sessions one of the other patient had befriended Bob and suggested that he try marijuana to help with his depression and it might help. Bob tried it and it help with his depression and he was able to continue his work on his job. He would take marijuana only on the occasion when he had heavy depression. Group therapy also was of great help to Bob with his recovery.

Anger Management

ANGER MANAGEMENT

Some people that have an anger management problem will take marijuana to calm their anger. Marijuana calms and relaxes them, as well for some it seems to make them happy and a bit passive. There are some people with this problem that are not where they even have a problem and if they know that they have an anger problem they will not admit it. There are many anger management classes and programs to help but some people have chosen to take this herbal medication to curb their anger. Anger can come in different degrees ranging from mild anger to rage. With the advent of more vehicles on the reads, road rage is on the rise affecting drivers in different degrees. Some times with some people the smallest thing cold set them off into an anger rage seemingly over nothing. Some people temper needs self control and calmness of the mind.

Testimonials - Anger Management, Mania and Mood Disorders

Kevin D. an AGGRESSION PROBLEM

Kevin D. has a anger management problem. Kevin is a 25year old electronics repairman that works in his father's electronics repair shop. Kevin would take medical marijuana to help his anger problem. For years Kevin had this problem with his temper. At times he would get so angry over what seems to be minor things of no consequence and for no real reason. It seemed that anything would make him angry For example if Kevin was waiting for the 3'00 o'clock train to arrive and if the train did not come on time at prissily at 3:00 he would start to become angry as the time moved on past 3:00. He would start to get angrier and angrier, as the minutes continued to pass minute by minute. He also has what's called borderline personality disorder. Kevin said that he would take medical marijuana to curb his moments of anger and relax him. He also would see a therapist to help him control his anger. Kevin is a very private person and would not give me too much information about the past 10 years of his experiences in the interview and I didn't press him about it. One thing you learn when interviewing a person is that has this disorder is not to aggravate the person or cause them stress. Aggravation or stress may trigger or set off a reaction with his type of disorder. Kevin might also have a Antisocial Personality Disorder. The therapist is making great progress with Kevin's treatment as well as teaching Kevin tolerance to others. Kevin is making good progress controlling his anger.

JACOB'S MOTHER'S TESTIMONIAL

When my son, Jacob, was a toddler he was easily frustrated. He couldn't even handle playing with blocks. If his blocks didn't set up right, he would pick them up and throw them around his room. By the time Jacob was three, he was destructive of his own property. He was so hard to control that my husband, Mel, and I thought something was wrong with him. Compared to our daughter, Carol, he was so much more aggressive. Our friends kept telling us, "Jacob is a boy. What do you expect? Boys are just more aggressive than girls." Even Jacob's doctor agreed. By the time he was four, Jacob was highly anxious about going to preschool. It would take me two hours to get him dressed, and then I had to physically put him on the school bus. When Jacob was five, he would assault other kids and he was destructive of himself to himself. It was horrendous. The first time my husband and I went to see a mental health professional, he told us that Jacob had separation anxiety because I had gone back to work after five years of being an at- home mom. He told me, "stop worrying, just give Jacob an extra hug every day and he'll be just fine." This same therapist kicked Jacob out of his office because he wasn't behaving properly! When Jacob was seven, he had a full-blown psychotic episode which lasted over five hours. He destroyed everything within sight, and we couldn't control him. My husband and I didn't know what to do. We didn't know how to access emergency services, and we didn't even know that such a thing as a crisis team existed. So we dealt with our son as best as we could. When Jacob finally collapsed with exhaustion. I picked up the phone and called a pastor in our community who also had a child with problems. I must have sounded like a mad woman on the phone, because the pastor and his wife met me at the church within twenty minutes. This was the first time I had ever connected with anyone who would cry with me and know exactly how I felt. Jacob's father and I went round and round searching for answers from one professional after another. We tried all kinds of techniques and every behavior modification program in the book to help our son. Nothing worked. After seeing our family for months, a child psychologist said to me " I can't do anything for you. You've done everything you can. This is about having a problem. Your son has bipolar disorder . This was the first time I understood that we weren't the worst parents in the world. I had repeated the story about Jacob to so many professionals by that time I had written a six- page report about his behavioral history. I gave it to the psychologist to look over, and then Jacob's father and I told her even more about Jacob's life. After about half an hour of listening to us. She said, "stop blaming yourselves. You didn't do this to Jacob. You've got a kid who has a mental illness. It's not your fault. It's not the end of the world. There's no cure, but there is treatment. It was so emotional to be told that your kid is sick, but it was probably one of the best days of my life. Most people wouldn't understand this, but because we finally had some answers, we could begin to see a path for working things out. Jacob was hospitalized a few days later so he could be stabilized. Jacob had never told me that he loved me until after his first hospitalization. He hadn't been able to get in touch with his emotional side enough to be able to express love. I'll never forget the day about two weeks after he came home from the hospital. I was doing the dishes and he came up behind me and said, "hey mom, I love you". I can't even describe how that felt. After that, he could say it a lot. He has began to share hugs more and more now.

I even get a happy little peck on the cheek. Our family used to have a super close friendship with our next door neighbors, but after Jacob's hospitalization, they went clean into the woodwork. It was the strangest thing I'd ever experienced in my life. Up until that time, we had the kind of relationship where we'd play cards together by the hour and have picnics together in our back yard. If Jacob had a major episode where he put a dent in their front door or something like that, I'd simply get a phone call and Jacob's father would go over and fix whatever Jacob had damaged. For some reason, Jacob's difficult behavior never put a strain on our friendship until he was diagnosed with a mental illness. At that point, they began to avoid us. I finally called my neighbor and said "come on over and let's chitchat over coffee. We haven't talked in a while." She came over and I put my feelings right out on the table. I said " what's going on? I don't understand the sudden change in our friendship." All she said was, "well we've just been real busy." It took me another six months before I finally figured out that they didn't want to be friends with our family anymore. Now, we just speak to them from a distance. This was very sad for me. People can be so ignorant about mental illness. On the other hand, my mother Jacob's grandmother has made a huge change in her attitude. This was a woman who used to talk about "crazy" people and make every ignorant statement about them that could possibly be made. Now when someone, says something negative about the mentally ill, my mother steps right up to bat and says, "just a minute, let me explain to you what mental illness really is." My mother has been transformed, and she has become incredibly supportive of Jacob and our family. I also have two brothers who live nearby, but we keep a kind of distance. We talk, but we don't talk about Jacob being sick. I choose not to make a major issue out of it. I don't drill knowledge about mental illness down anybody's throat if they aren't ready for it. By this time Jacob was fourteen years old and when he can home from his first hospitalization, we tried everything we could to help him. I gave up my full-time career in public relations because my life seemed so overwhelming. I felt like I needed to stay home and put the pieces of our lives back together. This put a pretty large hole in my personal plans and in my wallet, too, but I was convinced that it was the point where Jacob became my only life. I'd be with him all day long, and by the time Jacob's father came home from work, I was so fried that I just wanted to get out of the house and go for a walk. My husband would ask me to fill him in on what had been happening that day with Jacob and I'd give him a thirty second version of it as I walked out the door. There were also times when I would call my husband at work and say I can't do this anymore. I've had Jacob in restraints for forty-minutes, and he has unplugged every phone in the house and threatened to jump out the window. That was my life. Seeing other little boys about Jacob's age playing in the neighborhood made me feel resentful. It was just so unfair that my little guy didn't have that carefree, spontaneous life he was supposed to have at his age. We had a horrible time getting special education services for Jacob, because he was able to keep himself together pretty well in his school setting. He would contain his emotions all day and then he'd come home on a crazy, chaotic, noisy school bus and just explode the moment he came into the house.

Even if Jacob looked good to the school personnel, he rarely got past our front door before he would start up with oppositional behavior and aggressiveness. Jacob kept a journal in which he had written all kinds of suicide and homicidal notes while he was sitting in class. Even so, Jacob still got turned down for special services. I gave up. A year later, I said to myself I'm going back into the battle. In spite of, just when we got to the point where we started to win the fight with the school, Jacob was residential care. Our community just couldn't give our son what he needed at the time. And without enough community support, neither could we. Jacob is now eighteen and we put him in a residential treatment program was perhaps the hardest thing I've ever had to do. I knew it was the right thing for him and for the entire family, but that didn't make me feel any better about it. For the next couple of months, I found myself walking through my days feeling empty inside. It felt so painful, almost as if I had lost my son forever. Jacob has made tremendous progress in his residential treatment program. After three months there, he started to come home for visits. It was wonderful having him home again, but it took several months of visits before it didn't feel as if he were simply a guest in our house. Our family has healed and reconnected in a positive way. Jacob will be coming home soon to attend a community college. Our community mental health system did all that was possible but Jacob's school had just attended to his needs earlier. Jacob's roommate in college knew everything about his problems. He told Jacob he should try medical marijuana. Jacob was hesitant but his roommate was very pervasive and convincing. So Jacob tried the marijuana for a few days and he realized his roommate was right. It relaxed him and helped his mood swings and along with his medication he knew he had a good working combination. Jacob kept taking the marijuana and he never told his parents because he knew they wouldn't understand. He also knows that it is illegal to have marijuana in the State in which he lives, so he knows to be careful when buying it or taking it. Being bipolar means that I can get hyper real fast and aggressive, too and then I can become really depressed. Or I can be all of those things at the same time. But taking marijuana along with my meds helps me stay focused and do what my goals say I should do. It's getting easier to meet my goals thanks to medical marijuana, I have friends like I didn't have before. My illness can be treated and helped with medical marijuana, my other medication and therapy. I am maintaining thinks on a day to day basest and doing much better now.

Charles T. suffers from PERSONALITY DISORDER

Charles T. suffers from personality disorder, reactive depression and extended mood swings. Charles is an 26 year old computer programmer who is one of the top programmers in his field. Even though he's financially well off he has other problems and issues. Charles would complain of having night mares which would interrupt his sleeping pattern. For years he would go in and out of therapy sessions and counseling sessions which were ineffective for his needs. In the past he had a alcohol drinking problem in which every time he would drink alcohol to excess his personality would change in negative ways. He was like Dr. Jekyll and Mr. Hide, we all know that story. So he had to stop drinking alcohol all together. Charles would take marijuana which would inhibit his mood swings in such a way that they were controllable. It would help with his depression as well with his nightmares. He would say that when he had taken marijuana in the night time before bed he would not have nightmares. It would inhibit his dream pattern.

Debbie has been Charles's girlfriend for several years through good times and bad times. Debbie had noticed a difference in Charles. She noticed a change in Charles personality and attitude. He seem more calm and less stressed out. Charles slept better due to the absence of nightmares. Debbie noticed that he was much less critical on himself and go into a depressed state of mind that would last for day's and sometimes weeks. She also noticed that he was thinking in a different more positive outlook on life and a open mind when dealing with other matters. Debbie was happy when Charles had stopped drinking alcohol and is trying to put his life back together. Charles was eating better healthier foods and even exercising, feeling better about himself and thanking Debbie for staying with him during his trying times in the past. As Charles became mentally healthier and physically healthier, he began to make superior decisions with more confidence. We all live in what's called a cause and effect world, meaning one thing causes something else and effects it. Otherwise known as the domino effect. For Charles marijuana is not a cure but an aid that helps him deal with his sleep disorder, depression and mood swings. This worked for Charles where as this might not work for some others that have deeper mental problems and deeper issues.

William N has a form of MANIA

William N. has had a form of Mania all his life. He's now 57 years old but he acts like he's 27 years old. He always is the type of person that would do or try any type of physical activity such as sports, games, anything. Anything that was a thrill, he would do; Parachuting, skiing, hang gliding, fast cars, motor cycles, etc. There is nothing that's too dangerous that William wouldn't do. He always would become bored and restless wanting to do some activity. In many of his activities he fed off of the excitement and feeling that he could accomplish anything. In doing that he began to take to many chances and became reckless and dangerous to himself and others. He has had many accidents and broken bones but no one died. William has had many girlfriends but has never been married.

At the age of 57, William's body could no longer do all the things it used to do in the past. In other words, he realized that he was getting old and it was hard for him to except. Williams type of mania was mild and yet borderline. From all the injuries and broken bones throughout the years it finally took its toll with several types of arthritis. His doctors would prescribe several medications for the arthritis and mania. This mood disorder is not rare but rather common. The pain and discomfort of arthritis would be a constant reminder of William's age which he would not accept. He dealt with this by taking marijuana for the mania as well it helped him deal with the arthritis. Williams' type of mania is controllable so he could go through a normal daily situation and his mania was unnoticeable to others. But when a person got know him there was always something wrong. That's why he cannot keep a steady relationship with women. William would take the marijuana with other medication with no conflict or after effects. The marijuana would keep his moods of mania in check. High potency strains THC marijuana can have the effect of temporally appetite loss, as where low potency strains THC marijuana acts as a appetite inducer. Some people that have tested this theory out have said that when they smoke a high potency strain of marijuana it takes some time for an appetite to appear. Some people that take high potency THC strain say that they won't be hungry for an hour or two. Whereas the same people that will take low potency THC will get hungry in a half an hour. Some people say that high potency strains of marijuana are called sit down or lay down marijuana, because if you take too much of it, it makes you sit down or lay down. High potency strains of marijuana should be taken in small intervals to gradually increase the effect slowly. In this way they can limit its effect and instead of it being sit down or lay down marijuana, it becomes a pick me up type of marijuana. The pick me up type of marijuana has the effect of rejuvenating energy in the person at times.

Linda S. suffers from several MENTAL ILLNESSES

Linda S. is a 35 year old woman that suffers from several illnesses. Mania, Manic-depressive illness, and Mood-disorder. Linda was raised by a rich family that made her independently wealthy at a young age. Being able to have almost anything you wanted most of her life had made her very spoiled and not tolerant when not getting her way or what she wanted. When things did not go Linda's way or according to her plans she would become manic-depressive. One minute she would be very depressed then switch to anger which would become vindictive and spiteful. When in this state of mind Linda would go on a buying stress or travel as if to relieve the disappointment by doing purchases which made her feel better. Having been married for a short time and divorced soon after with no children Linda found herself alone and unhappy. She was having difficulty in having relationships with the men she was seeing. Linda's selfishness and attitude always stood in the way. She had been always raised as a princess or a queen that she was expecting to have a prince or a king. Linda was looking for Mr. perfect as a spouse but as we all know that no one is perfect and you have to settle for less than perfect or you will stay alone for a long time. One day when Linda was driving to the store she got into a minor car accident in the store parking lot which was clearly her fault and yet she would deny it. The person she had the accident with was Bruce T. an employee of a car dealership. For Linda it was love at first site as if he was the one man she always wanted. As for Bruce he was less than impressed with Linda's superior attitude and was not attracted to her because of it. They exchanged information for insurance purposes and left. By no means did their life styles match or were they compatible. They were almost opposites and yet Linda didn't seem to care. As far as she was concern he was the one for her. Bruce was a struggling sales man that lives a somewhat boring life of a 9 to 5 employee. Bruce's idea of spending a nice week end is to sleep late, watch sports games on the TV set, going fishing or working with one of his many hobbies or projects. Were as Linda would do a lot of traveling to different places in search of something to fill a void in her life. Linda had masked Bruce out to go to a movie and Bruce said, alright. After their first date Bruce knew that they were incompatible as a couple and yet he was still attracted to her. He knows that she is not his type of woman that he likes and thinks they live in two different worlds and that this first date would probably be there last date. Linda knew that the first date did not go well because of herself. She was smart enough to see that the problem was with herself as in all her past relationships.

Whereas Linda had similar reservations about having a relationship with Bruce but she had fell in love with Bruce and realized that she really loved someone more than here self. She was determined that he was not going to walk out of her life without a major effort to win his love. So she decided to work on herself and major problems which she had ignored but was aware of such mania. She would go to a psychiatrist and take light medications such as medical marijuana which relaxed her and made her think in a different way and analyze things more open minded to make better decisions. After about 4 weeks Linda called up Bruce to set up a date. At first Bruce didn't think a second date would have been any different from their first date but Linda had convinced him to go out on a second date. On the second date Linda was like a totally different person. She wasn't arrogant, spoiled, or rude. She was considerate, pleasant, and open minded. The very opposite of their first date. At first Bruce thought it was just and act and that a person can't change in such a short period. He couldn't believe that she was the same woman. so he asked her to go on a third date. This made Linda smile and happy. Linda decided to change her way of thinking and attitude. She had learned that the old saying that you get more bees with honey than you do with vinegar. On their third date it was even better than the second date, and they got to know each other better and realized they both would have to make changes with themselves. They both would have to make compromises with each other. Sometimes opposites attract and do work out. Linda would continue to go to her therapist and take medication and learn more about herself and about others. As time moved on Bruce and Linda became more of an item even though they have their differences they learn to adapt to each other and Bruce soon fell in love with Linda. Linda's family noticed the change in Linda's attitude and personality and were happy about the change in her. To them she was pleasant to be around and they began to invite her to all the family functions. Linda had never really been in love with any one before including her first husband. So for her this was worth any changes or sacrifice on her part to make the relationship work. She learned how to control her mania with medical marijuana medication as a mental relaxer and therapy.

Edna A has MANIC EPISODES

Edna A. is 28 years old and has had manic episodes (mania, mood disorder) most of her life. Edna is a pretty woman that works for the Banking System. She lives alone and really does not have any friends. Edna is the type of person that thinks they are smarter than everyone else or better than everyone else. She tries to make friends with others but she always puts her foot in her mouth by saying something wrong. Sometimes her thoughts just rush out of her mouth before thinking about what she is saying. She alienates people away from her. Edna thinks that the other people in the banking office are slow moving, boring, and stupid and that there is something wrong with them, but it is her. Edna would get irritable in the blink of an eye and her mood would change and then change back. It seemed very important for her to think that she is the best of the best in all her endeavors. Edna always has a answer for everything which may be incorrect at times. She has sleeplessness and yet still has energy to do her daily work. Edna has seen many doctors throughout the years for her mania. Sometimes Edna's thoughts race in her mind where she losses thought of the original idea.

Edna takes marijuana which relaxes her mind and in doing so she can concentrate on one thing at a time. Edna realizes that the problem is not in others but in herself. Then she feels lonely and depressed. And then she realizes that she has to change the way she is thinking and slow it down so she could concentrate on one thing at a time and learn patience. Edna wou7ld take marijuana at home in the place of the martini drink in the evening. The marijuana also helped Edna with her sleeping problem by letting her sleep normal hours. Edna is a good worker at her job but her fellow workers think that she is strange or wacky. That would soon change and the other workers would except her. Edna is changing the way she thinks about things and Edna has a long way to go.

Testimonials - Stress
Linda and Rick have problems with STRESS
Linda and Rick have been married for 8 years. Linda is Swedish and was brought up a devout Catholic in the outskirts of Stockholm. Rick is Jewish and lived in several large Eastern cities while growing up. Linda was pregnant when she got married and converted as a condition of the marriage. Both Linda and Rick are in their early 30's, but both had been told though out their adult lives that they were infertile. When Linda became pregnant, they were both over joy and both decided to get married. They had a son and within 10 months of the first child they had a set of twin boys as well. Their troubles began some 11 months prior to seeking treatment when Linda developed a terrible case of cystitis. She felt constant pressure on her bowel and had to urinate every 15 to 30 minutes. Her tests kept coming back "negative" and she was told it was probably stress related. The problem got much worse whenever they had sex. Linda began to get very nervous whenever she wasn't

near a bathroom. She avoided any physical contact with Rick lest he wanted to have sex with her. Rick was supportive for the first 6 or 7 months. Then he began worrying about whether they were ever going to have sex again. Rick felt that Linda had become self absorbed and obsessed about the cystitis. She no longer was interested in what was happening with him. Often she would break into tears while lying in bed or watching TV. She kept on saying that Rick couldn't understand and that she needed to be alone. Rick started to withdraw and have a cool, removed manner. Linda felt that it was the beginning of the end of her marriage and she had to do something. Eventually Rick acknowledged his own drinking problem. Rick was forced to face his own addiction. They had financial problems and they were quickly slipping into bankruptcy. Linda was trying to work with the lawyers without Rick's help. Rick slept a lot and usually had nightmares, he was uninterested in doing any couple activities. Linda wanted to make things right with Rick. She loved him deeply and was totally committed to the marriage. She was frustrated that although seemed to make it right, Rick also professed deep love and commitment for Linda. However he did not label himself as depressed. He said he was always a serious and quiet person. This had always been a problem between him and Linda. He felt he was justified to feel this way about his life. He agreed he was a terrible husband but was unable to follow through on any suggestions for increased participation in his marital life. Linda's optimism was the catalyst for getting married and having children. Being around Linda was evicting and interesting. Within a short time, Rick began to feel pressured to be someone that he knew he would never be. Linda was a night person and Rick was a morning person who liked jogging during the early day break hours. Rick began to feel that the personality differences between them were unbridgeable. Linda did too much, talked too much, and thought too much for him.

The first treatment consisted of Rick's drinking problem. He went to A.A. twice, sometimes three times a week. Linda was an exercise instructor and personal trainer. She worked with many different people. She was very resourceful, optimistic, willing to listen, filled with ideas for activities, and able share in an intimate and open matter. The most important parts of therapy were the joint marital therapy sessions. After a few sessions, two main marital issues emerged. Rick's long buried resentments over Linda's assumption that he would be the primary bread winner and Linda's feeling that his private and quietness were passive aggressive maneuvers to get back at her. Over the course of several sessions, Linda admitted that for many years she had relied on Rick to financially support the family but realized that in the future they would have to share that burden. She related her dependency on Rick to a desire to have the security she never felt as a child growing up in a chaotic, abusive, alcoholic home. Rick began to see how he had to give Linda some clear clues as to what he was feeling so that she wouldn't interpret his withdrawal as a personal attack. Linda starts eating organics, educates herself about natural herbs and supplements. She changes her lifestyle, includes herbs and supplements in her diet, she tries marijuana and three months later a marked improvement . The cystitis was gone and so were the panic attacks. Therapy lasted 6 months and there able to enjoy some time together and work on family issues together. By the end of therapy and with the help of medical marijuana Rick's depression and nightmares had lifted and he found a job with a well established company at a good salary. He was much more optimistic and was able to think more clearly. Their sex problems were dealt with by having them enjoy sex for a period of weeks. They started using a condom when they were having sex. The problem got under control whether it was due to sex or something else was unclear. Linda had mentally decided to take whatever precautions she could and then enjoy her sex life.

Grace suffers from STRESS

It was obvious that Grace being a young inexperienced mother of three small children was becoming overwhelmed with all the differences and new facets and responsibility that she has. The stress began to affect her physically and mentally. Grace would begin to loss patients with the children more frequently and become stressed out. She began to not eat properly, lose weight and lose interest in her own survival and concentrate on what she thought was more important which was her responsibility to her family. She began to become sickly due to a low resistance because of lack of proper nutrients in her body. This made Grace more susceptible to colds and other germs. Grace's husband Fred noticed the difference in his wife and would help out with the children and house duties to aid his wife. Fred still has to work a 9 to 5 job so he only could help out after work and on the weekends which was a great help to his wife. Grace had remembered when she was in high school and back in the days when she would hang out and what was called party a lot. She remembered when she smoked marijuana and how it had calmed her nerves and relieved her stress especially when she had finals in high school. Grace also remembered that marijuana had gave her a veracious appetite for food. She thought of how she could tell her husband Fred what she wanted to do. To try marijuana to see if it could help her with her stress and appetite. Grace also tells him and does so, he naturally has a negative response to her idea and said no to it. But after a few days he changed his mind and did what Grace wanted. This was not easy for Fred to do or did he want to but he loves his wife and wanted to please her so he contacted a few of his friends to buy some marijuana for Grace.

After all, it's not like Fred could just go down to the local pharmacy with a prescription for medical marijuana. Fred got the marijuana and gave it to Grace under certain conditions and stipulations. She would never smoke it around the children and only smoke it outside the house or in her bathroom with the window open. After about two weeks Fred saw a change in Grace for the better. She seem less up tight and stressed out at the end of the day and she was eating more food. She was more active with the children and in her own life. After several months Grace was back at her correct weight for her age and height and her stress became a thing of the past. She would soon stop taking marijuana and no longer take it for the stress problem and weight problem.

Phobias

There are hundreds of different phobias that affect millions of people every day. These fears are from the mental psyche an can be treated in different ways. Phobias can be beaten with knowledge of a fear an learning why the person has the fear of a particular phobia and dealing with it. Marijuana has been used as a mild relaxer medication, to relax the phobic person's mind. Everyone has had stress some time in their life. Some people hardly ever have stress and then others have stress on a daily bases. There are different degrees of stress levels from low to high stress levels. The most common stress can be caused by ones job or life style or problems affecting ones mental condition. Stress can also affect ones physically with chemical changes. The term stressed out is frequently used which means at the maximum level.

Testimonials - Phobias and Panic Disorders

Peter E suffers from ANHEDONIA

Peter E. is suffering from Anhedonia (loss of pleasure due to major depression). Recently Peter's older brother was killed in the war and it had devastated Peter emotionally. The psychological trauma plunged Peter into major depression. Peter has gone through changes in most aspects of his life at the age of 24. Peter's depression affects his motivation, thinking, and physical and motor functioning. Peter felt despair, unhappiness, frequent crying spells. He shows signs of loss of interest of pleasure. The things that Peter liked to do he lost interest in doing. Whether it is going over a friend's house or playing a video game or playing in sports activities. He has lost interest in the pleasures he use to do. He lost body weight from not eating food due to the depression. He has insomnia, awakening too early and can't go back to sleep. He's caught up in a cycle of cause and effect. He's taken off many day's from work and about to be laid off from his job and he does not seem to care. Peter also shows signs of irritable and anger over his brother's death. Peter's girlfriend, named Sue noticed right away there was something wrong with Peter's attitude and thinking. Sue suggested that he get help for his depression. Peter knew that there was something wrong with himself but didn't want to seek help for fear of being labeled as a person that has mental problems. He was afraid that if he went to a therapist he would have a record of having mental problems. Sue convinced Peter to get help from a professional therapist that specialized in major depression. Sue would go with Peter to some of the talk therapy sessions which were helping greatly. Peter would be prescribed medications for the depression which he did not like. He said the medication made him feel doped up and groggy and he stopped taking it. One day Sue came over to Peter's house with some marijuana for Peter with the hope that this would help him sleep through the night and as a appetite inducer. At first Peter didn't want to try it but after a short time Sue had convinced Peter to smoke some of the marijuana before he went to bed. That night Peter smoked a little bit of the marijuana before bed time and went right to sleep. The next morning Peter got up after sleeping for 8 hours straight through the night without interruption. That morning Sue stopped by Peter's house before going to work to check on Peter and found him in the kitchen making breakfast. Sue was in shock seeing Peter making breakfast because he would always skip breakfast. Sue asked Peter, how are you feeling this morning? Peter said, I feel fine but I'm starving. I feel like I haven't eaten in a day so I'm making something to eat. Would you like to have some? Sue said, no thank you, with a smile I have to go to work and I'll see you later. Before Sue went out the door she turned and said to Peter. How did you sleep last night? Peter said, I slept straight through the night. Sue said, good and left. As Sue was walking she thought to herself, the marijuana had worked. Peter slept through the night and had an appetite as well. From that day on, Peter would take marijuana as a sleep inducer and appetite stimulus. Peter still would go to therapy sessions and begin to go back to his old self. Peter began to be more optimistic and hopeful in his thinking. He was sleeping better and his body weight started to increase back to normal. He would soon go back to work once again.

Roger L. suffers from a PANIC DISORDER

Roger L. is a 27 year old male who was referred to case management by the psychiatric hospital treatment staff because of a history of symptoms of panic disorders which include palpitations, sweating, feelings of choking, chest pain, feeling dizzy, fear of losing control and psychotic features. Given the research into biological aspects of panic disorder, several insights are important to Rogers case. Panic and other anxiety disorders have a strong family contribution, these individuals whose family members have these disorders are at increased risk of developing these disorders. Medications proscribed by a physician may be helpful in changing the neurochemistry associated with Roger's panic symptoms. Roger was first hospitalized at age 18, during what was diagnosed as a manic episode while he was a community college student. Roger had parked his car on the freeway one night when he ran out of gas, and walked several miles to the airport. He was taken to the hospital by the police, who had been called by airport security to respond to Rogers bizarre behavior in the airport terminal.

Roger has been on medication since that time and he has been seeing a psychiatrist at a county outpatient mental health clinic. He was diagnosed with panic disorder with psychotic features. Roger has not resumed going to community college. He lives with his parents and three older siblings in a single family home. His parents have been reluctant to permit the intervention of mental health professionals. They tend not to seek help until Roger becomes unmanageable and out of control, at which time his behavior often attracts the attention of the police. Roger was very cooperative during the initial interview at his home. He signed consent forms to enable the case manager to obtain information from his father and sister Anna who have taken the roles of mental health professionals. The case manager watches Roger interactions with family members, talks with Roger about his interests and briefly discuss the effect of his illness on himself and his family. Roger shows no insight into his problems. He doesn't relate well and states that people overreact, to him. When asked about past incidents leading to police involvement, Roger laughs and says, but I was only acting! Roger's medications are stored in a cabinet in the kitchen, where several out dated bottles are mixed in with current prescriptions. With assistance Roger sorts through the bottles and safely disposes of the old medication by flushing the pills. The case manager provides a pill organizer and helps Roger organize medication into individual compartments, taken daily for a full week.

This will lessen Roger's confusion about the correct dosages and enable the case manager to monitor his medication by counting what remains of the current supply. Roger's sister provides his case manager with additional information about her brothers current and past functioning, including his occasional uncontrolled spending sprees. Roger's father is currently trying to clear up bills for expensive gold jewelry and a health club membership purchased by his son. Roger does not know his monthly income and cannot name any expenses he has other than buying an occasional soda from the local market. Roger's father gives him small amounts of money whenever he asks for it. Most of the excessive spending has been the result of Roger getting instant credit for purchases. Roger's case manager scheduled a meeting with him to discuss his goals for the next six months. The meeting was held at his home. Roger wanted to resume his education in computer assisted design at the local community college.

Roger was agreeable to having assistance with medication but was offended by the case manager's characterization of his spending problem. Roger stated he was open to learning more about his income and expenses since his father currently handled all his money. Roger stated he wanted to work on getting his own apartment. Although this was a reasonable goal Roger's sister explained that it was unacceptable in the Filipino culture, where you stay with the family until you get married. For this reason and because the case manager wanted to gain the families trust and cooperation this goal was deferred. A couple of weeks later Roger runs into an old friend Sean he hasn't seen in five years at a bus stop. They agree to meet up on the weekend, they catch up on old times and Roger tells him about his situation Sean tells him about medical marijuana and how it helped his anxiety, stress and depression. Roger tried it, almost instantly he felt relief. So much so that he could go back to community college six months later with the help of medical marijuana he was on his way to finishing and getting his degree.

Testimonials - Mental Illnesses and Other Disorders

Jody R. has a history of MENTAL ILLNESS

My name is Jody R. and I don't think I can even describe to anybody what it's like to be mentally ill. I've been mentally ill since I was a little girl. I've not been able to live at home since I was thirteen, and I will probably never to function outside of a highly structured environment. I live with full time staff and two others in a little house on the grounds of a residential treatment facility in Philadelphia. When I think on all the years that I was psychotic, I can't believe that my family got through those times and came out the other side. Now that I am doing so much better, it's tempting to think that it wasn't that bad. But it was that bad. It was a night mare for my entire family, but especially for me. Thanks to medical marijuana and my meds it changed my life for the better. By the time I was ten, I was walking around with a sense of dread. That feeling has never completely gone away even though I'm thirty years old now. In my childhood years, I didn't seem to take in information the way that I should. It was obvious that at the very least I had severe learning disabilities, but I always sensed some sort of emotion al confusion. I was fragile and extremely anxious. When I was fifteen I got hit by a car while my family was on vacation in Florida. I had no head injuries, thank God, but I spent months in traction at a local hospital. My mom brought me home by train because I was encased in a heavy, plaster full body cast. When my cast was finally removed two months later, I was terrified of the outdoors, of odors, of any sudden noise and even the wind. I was so frightened I really couldn't function outside of the house. My mom suspected that my emotional difficulties weren't caused just by the car accident. She believed that I was suffering from more than post-traumatic stress disorder. I saw a child psychologist twice a week for the next three years. This woman was very honest with my mother. She felt that I would probably never be able to lead a completely normal life, and that she would always need structure and psychiatric help. By the time I was seven or eight I began to show clear signs of mental illness. I would wash my hands compulsively until they were raw and bleeding, I would stand in front of the mirror for hours on end to make sure that my eyes were in the right place on my face. I was very reluctant to go outside because I thought that flies and even bits of grass would enter my body and damage me in some way. My mother would always be worried about how my day went at school, sometimes I would be so unsettled that the entire evening would be ruined. The smallest things would set me off. And it would take me hours to settle down again. If I misplaced something, even a tiny thing, everybody in the family would have to stop what they were doing immediately and look for it.

Shortly before I turned thirteen my parents couldn't take care of me at home anymore. I was admitted to a psychiatric hospital on an emergency basis. My mother couldn't find the words to explain to me why I could no longer live at home. The situation was also very hard on my younger brother. One particular day about fifteen years ago I was home on a pass. My mother and I were shopping downtown. I could sense my anxiety level was building rapidly. I ran away from my mother and she couldn't catch up with me.

I ran screaming down the street. A policeman helped me chase her, calling for back-up. A squad car finally cornered her in a parking garage, and one cop straddled her because she was so out of control. The worst of it was that the police assumed that I was on it was that the police assumed that I was on drugs. They threw me in their car any way and took her to the emergency room, where she was finally stabilized hours later. I can talk about this episode now with a sense of detachment but for many years afterword I wasn't comfortable with anybody who wore a uniform. Just thinking about this incident is still unbearably painful.

In the early years of my illness, my friends would often ask about me. But when I left home to live in residential treatment centers and various locked inpatient psychiatric units, the news about me was usually so grim that after a while a lot of them how much pain I was in. There are so many myths about the various treatments for mental illness. I have had over twenty electroshock treatments, each one was easy, quick and painless. When I was in my twenties I had two neurosurgical operations. My anxiety decreased dramatically and thanks to medical marijuana my life was worth living. One thanksgiving when I was about eighteen, the entire family was sitting around talking about current events and I totally lost control. I ended up in the emergency room. I think that's what happened when I realized that my brothers were two grown men who led normal lives. I took so many years of energy from my mom even though my mom's been there for me forever. She calls me all the time, she advocates for me. I may have severe psychiatric problems, but if I'm having a good day I can be fabulous. I have a great sense of humor and sensitivity to others. I can deal with my symptoms now in a better way. I no longer get aggressive or psychotic like I did when I was younger. I used to throw things, hurt myself or break windows out of frustration and terror. My mom and dad write and call me often. I like hearing from them and being with them. My life used to be scary and difficult, and sometimes it still is. But I know how to handle the rough times now. This makes me feel happy and proud of myself. For the most part, people have been kind to me. But some people have been mean to me by teasing me and being rude and making fun of me. I wish I had never gotten sick. Maybe I could have gone to college. I'm thankful that I'm much better now and that I have mostly recovered from my hard times. But I don't like living away from home. I miss my family. I'm happy that I come home a lot and that I can travel with my family to our other home in Idaho. I also have friends now and a dog who lives with me in my house. Sometimes I'm unhappy because I haven't had an easy life. My brothers can do more than me, but someday maybe I can do some of the things they can, like driving a car and be more independent. I'm starting to do some of the things that my brothers do, like use a computer. I even have a job. I'm mostly all better now. I used to be depressed and scared and anxious and I didn't love myself. I love myself now. I'm a good person and thankful for being me. I know that my positive qualities come from my parents and all they have done for me over the years. I also try to look on the best side of things. I once read that more money is spent on research for Schizophrenia. These priorities don't seem right to me. The issue of mental illness must be raised to the level of a national problem so that appropriate funds used to help. Not many people can afford good medical care.

Charles S. suffers from MULTIPLE ILLNESSES

Charles S. has been diagnosed with depression, attentional problems, learning disabilities, diabetes and family stress. Charles is 23 years old man who feels isolated, depressed and hopeless. He goes to Community College. He has few friends, his school work is poor and he feels uncomfortable in his predominately Caucasian College. He's new at school, recently moving to a new town from out of state. He constantly complains that he doesn't fit in He was evaluated by a psychologist and was found to experience an attentional problems as well as a learning disability that makes reading difficult.

He has taken medication in the past for his attentional problems and also takes insulin for his diabetes. Charles mother works as a social worker at a local hospital. She was recently diagnosed with breast cancer. His father works as a clerk in a large computer company. His mother is Catholic and very active in her Church where as his father describes himself as an atheist. His father has had an alcoholism problem for many years and has suffered from depression as well. He has been fired from many jobs due to his alcohol troubles and temper. Charles parents have had a great deal of marital conflict and have separated on several occasions. Their differences in faith, ethnic background, financial concerns, and temper have taken a toll on the family. Charles younger sister is a "star" student, that has a lot of friends, and seems to cope very well the stress in the family Charles feels that his sister makes him look bad. Charles is willing to get help but feels that there is little any one can do for him.

One day while he was eating lunch a classmate sat down next to him and they started to talk. Charles told his classmate everything he was going through. He needed to tell someone even though he had some trust issues. His classmate told him he should try some marijuana. Charles was skeptical but he felt he should try it. The next day his classmate brought Charles some marijuana. Charles went home and smoked the marijuana and immediately he felt calm and relaxed. As time moved on the marijuana helped Charles with his depression, attentional problems and family stress as well as his prescribed medication. Even though Charles know it's risky buying marijuana but it's made his life better. Charles began to improve more each day. The marijuana helped in conjunction with his other medications.

Brandie M. suffering from HYPERTHYROIDISM

Brandie M. is 25 years old and suffering from Hyperthyroidism. Brandie's thyroid gland produces to any hormones in her causing her anxiety, stress, weight loss, weakness. Brandie is a model that appears in advertising billboard pictures, magazines, TV commercials, and walking down ramps in fashion shows. Brandie approaching the top in her field as a model when she was diagnosed with hyperthyroidism. Brandie would always watch her weight not thinking that there was anything wrong with herself. She was not aware that she had a thyroid gland problem. At one of the fashion shows that Brandie was a part of she had fainted due to lack of energy and weakness. At first her doctors thought that she was suffering from anorexia nervosa because of her low weight and the nature of her profession. But that was not the case. After going to several different doctors had tested and examined her diagnosed with Hyperthyroidism. She was prescribed medication to lower her hormone production and anxiety medications. The thyroid gland effects many important organs in the body. Being hat we live in a cause and effect world, our bodies work the same way. One thing causes and effects something else. Brandie didn't like taking the anxiety medication so she sort other types of anxiety medications and tried marijuana for her anxiety. She found that it had helped her feel better and relaxed with no after effects. She also found that the marijuana had increased her appetite which was an added benefit for her. Brandie's boy friend would supply the marijuana for her and she would take it along with the other prescribed medications. Brandie use to have some of these symptoms, heart racing, hands sweating, faint or dizzy, weakness and unable to relax. These symptoms have subsided for now. Brandie has put on healthy body weight due to the increase in appetite as well as an increase in energy output on her part.

Samantha T. suffering from MENTAL TRAUMA

Samantha T. is a 25 year old that is suffering from the trauma of being raped by a stranger. It had left her in a fearful state of mind and not trusting others especially men. She felt responsible and guilt for what had happened which was not her fault. Samantha is a victim of a crime. She has emotional problems, such as low self-esteem, depressed mood, antisocial actions. Sexual problems, intimacy problems and a fear of future victimization. Samantha receives specialized rape counseling services from the rape crisis center and hot line. The professional individual support for Samantha as well as group sessions. Center volunteers help her through the procedures and assisted her with any legal red tape and advocated in her behalf. It has been two years since Samantha was attacked and has left her with long term effects in the form of phobias. Samantha has made some progress with her problems but she needs more time. She is still not socializing the way she would in the past. She is still not dating men, the way she use to. Not that she was not asked out to socialize, but she was asked out to socialize many times by different men. She would continue to see a therapist and take medications that were prescribed. Samantha didn't like taking sleeping pills so she would take marijuana a half hour before bed time to help her sleep straight through the night without the usual night mares that she would have. After about six months Samantha was slowly getting her life back together. One day Samantha's old school friend Gail called her and invited her over for a little birthday dinner, and would not take no for an answer. So Samantha promised to go to the birthday dinner not knowing that Gail also invited a man named Patrick to come to. Gail was playing match maker which she always liked to do with much success in matching the correct pair of people. Gail had hoped that Samantha and Patrick might be attracted to each other and that they have a lot in common. Gail was playing match maker and setting up a double date dinner. The night of the dinner when Samantha arrived and saw that there was just the four of them, she knew that Gail had set her up to meet a man. As for Patrick he knew that Gail was setting them up on a double date. He had seen Samantha before and he liked what he saw. Samantha at first was not to happy that she had been set up by her friend in a position that she was unprepared for, but Samantha would hold her temper and play along with it. When Patrick was introduced to Samantha he was happy to finely meet her after seeing her around the area and wanting to meet her. With Patrick it was love at first site and he had made up his mind that Samantha was the one for him. Even though he knew nothing about her he was willing to learn about her and win her over.

Samantha seem to be attracted to him but a bit stand offish. The dinner went well and Samantha gave Patrick her phone number so they could talk and get to know each other. Patrick called up Samantha several time before they went out on a date to the movies. Patrick is not the type of man to pressure a woman for sex, he's a real gentleman that's looking for a long term relationship possibly marriage. The movie date went well and they found out that they had a lot in common as well as a lot of differences which made for a good match. After the end of the date Samantha invited Patrick into her apartment for tea or coffee. While they drank the tea Samantha lit up a joint of marijuana and offered it to Patrick. Patrick said, I don't smoke but you go right ahead. Samantha explained why she smokes marijuana because of her problem with insomnia and body weight loss but stopped short of telling him about being attacked. They seem to be getting along well although Samantha was still stand offish. Samantha will tell Patrick about the attack but that was not the right time to do so. Patrick is a nice, understanding man that's falling in love with Samantha and her dark past would not have any effect on the way he feels about her.

Paula G. suffers from a MENTAL ILLNESS

My name is Paula G., I come from a middle-class African- American family, and I believe that my parents tried to do the things for me that they thought were important. My mother would take me to plays and stuff like that but it seemed like the moment I got a little bit older, a lot of the good stuff she did for me just stopped. I didn't get the proper nurturing that a child should get. My mother even refused to hug me. She was emotional abusive, which did a lot of damage to my self-esteem. I didn't do well in school because there were always problems at home. My parents fought all the time, and my home life was chaotic. My mother was constantly out of control. She was a very good school teacher, but not so good a parent. When I was twelve I began to have nightmares every night. I was a big Kennedy fan, and I read a lot about the J.F.K. assassination. There was always something on TV about it that I would watch. I had a bit of a fixation about it. I would dream that I was riding in the motorcade with the president when he was killed. I would watch the president's head get blown off and I'd wake up screaming. The TV news cast of the assassination was not seen until years after but it was just as I had dreamt it. I've been scared all of my life. I was a very sickly child, which didn't help my social skills. I didn't have any friends. I was just plain afraid of people. I was very quiet at school never saying a word. I just kind of sunk in and became numb with no facial expression or emotion. I hardly ever laughed. I stood out because I was so different. When you have problems, kids pick up on it. They saw that I wasn't any good at academics or sports. I had nothing that they could see to respect. I was working down the street once and a bunch of girls started throwing rocks at me. They began to tease me about my African features, and what really hunted me was that they were black children. I became afraid of my own people! When I was in the sixth grade, my teacher called my mother complaining about some problems. My mother took me to a clinic where I met with a black female psychologist. I looked at her and was scared to death. For one thing she was kind of hard. I think she really was trying to reach out to me, but I was too far gone. This psychologist would take me out and I wanted to run. She kept trying to work with me but I wanted out, I wanted to get away from this woman. She said if I didn't get away from this woman. She said if I didn't get help now everything would go downhill. I didn't listen to my psychologist and I quit therapy. Later on, I went to a child guidance center and backed away from that too. My mother never insisted upon it or anything. I just got the hell out of there because I was afraid. By the time I was a teenager, I had all of this anger inside of me. I had nothing inside of me that I respected. One of the worst years of my life was when I was seventeen. I ran out my classes at high school because I was so frightened of people. My classmates teased me. They didn't understand me because I had problems with my sexual identity. I'm not saying that I'm gay, but there

83

was some confusion there. They used to call me asexual, homosexual, everything in the book. I did have four girlfriends who stuck by me, and I'm sure glad of that.   I graduated high school by the skin of my teeth. After graduation, I went to a community college. Because I no longer had the closeness of my four high school friends any more. I was walking through junior college with nobody.

I went downhill emotionally. My mother saw me lying in a fetal position one day, and the next thing I knew she took me to a psychiatric ward down in Los Angeles. She told me if I don't get myself together then this was the way I would end up. That place scared the hell out of me. The people in there were very, very sick. I think my mother was trying, in her own way to stop something, but she basically scared me out of my mind. When I was twenty-one, I went to live in a board- and – care apartment because the professors at my college could see that I really needed help. It was scary for me to leave home. That's when I began my journey of being an African American in the mental health world. I went to a clinic where I was diagnosed with major depression and anxiety. A psychiatrist there began medicating me with all different types of drugs. I was medicated to the point where I was a zombie. I became known as the weird person, my family all backed away from me, which really hurt. I developed agoraphobia. I would go out at night so nobody could see me. All my other girlfriends turned away from me. Five years ago I was gravely disabled and homeless. I began walking through the city at 2:00a.m., hearing voices twenty-four hours a day telling me what to do. The voices got to the point of my wanting to kill myself. When I got out of this hospital, I remember lying down on the street and hoping a car would run me over, so I could stop hearing the voices in my head. Over the years, I've lived in several different board-and-care apartments. I was the first person to move in there, and I was also one of very few African Americans in the neighborhood. The problem was a lot of white men started moving into the board-and-care. They were mentally ill too, but they all accepted me. However, the neighbors began to spread rumors about me because I was friends with these young white guys. I became known as the prostitute of the neighborhood because I was black and walking with white guys it got to the point where I became really,

really paranoid. I was afraid of people and don't trust them. Now something happened to reinforce what I felt. I'm most proud of the fact that I didn't commit suicide, and I do smoke marijuana which has helped me do things I couldn't do before, it's helped me socialize, relax and remain calm. I want to be the Harriet Tubman who bring not just my people, but all people to the side of good mental health. I wanted to help other mentally ill people get to the point where they can live as comfortable as possible. I want to be able to reach people so I can really make a difference. I think my people are going to have to learn to speak up more. A lot of therapy they automatically think "crazy". But I also think other races may have this belief, too. But I've been around my people and I know they say this stuff. They're not comfortable in revealing things about themselves. When you say a person is nothing but a schizophrenic, it's an insult. It's almost like saying a cuss word, it's like saying "all black people eat watermelon". All mentally ill people don't go out and murder people. Most mentally ill people are not violent they are into their own world. Did the mental health system fail me? In some ways, yes it did. The professionals should have set more boundaries and limits with me, but it's really up to us as people with mental illness to get up and fight.

And that's what I've begun doing. All the things that I've been through, even though they were painful, have shaped me to become a person I respect. I'm going back to school to become a counselor, because I truly care about people. I've been told that I have a gift with people. I know how to address them. When it's needed, I know how to comfort them. Medical marijuana has helped me leave my apartment and relaxed me to be able to speak in public. It's helped me calm down enough to get my thinking where it's slow enough for me to verbalize whatever I want to say. I've decided not to have children because I'm afraid they might be mentally ill like me. I don't want any child of mine going into an institution. I plan to live a good life. I'd like to step out and have fun at this point in my life. And that's something that I never could have said before. If you don't respect yourself, you get stepped on. I got stepped on a lot. Now I'm learning to respect myself. That's just the way life can be.

TESTIMONIALS

When I was a junior in High School, I was diagnosed with clinical depression. Every day living turned into a challenge for me. Things as simple as eating or getting dressed in the morning were difficult, much less having the concentration to do my school work. Given what I know now about depression, my symptoms could have been creeping up on me as early as elementary school. From the fourth grade on, I experienced extreme emotional swings and an unusually strong attachment to certain people. My mother had to take me to work with her because I was emotionally out of control. I left home to go to boarding school in the ninth grade. Soon after I arrived, I went through to waves of bad depression and I had trouble eating and sleeping. In my sophomore years, I had my first breakdown. I was in a diving meet. When I made my first dive and didn't do it perfectly. I totally lost it. I started to cry and I couldn't stop. When I went back to my dorm that night. I still couldn't pull myself back together.

The next week was exam week, and my mother had to come take me home because I was falling apart. Luckily my teachers let me take my exams at home. I returned to school when the exam period ended, and I was able to complete the year. In my junior year, I was in trouble from the start. Once again, I had difficulty eating and sleeping. I was living in a dorm, but I isolated myself from my peers. I didn't go out, and I spent most of my time alone. I was ashamed because I thought that my feelings of depression were caused by a lack of strength or will on my part. I wanted to suck it up and get through by myself. I broke down again during exam week just as I had the year before. When I had to leave school a second time, the staff said, "this issue has to be addressed". They referred me to a psychiatrist, who diagnosed me with clinical depression. I felt like I was finally being taken care of. The school had stepped in. It was out of my hands, and I was relieved because I didn't have to manage everything on my own anymore. Once my school got involved, I felt like I could let myself go and just be me. School became a safety net that was there to catch me. I only told two other people besides my mother and my therapist about my situation. One was a girl that had gone to my school the years before and the other was one of my teachers. They were both incredibly good listeners and very supportive. They didn't try to "fix me". They simply let me be me and say what I wanted to say.

You can be irrational when you're depressed, and they understood that. After I was diagnosed, I was put on medication. I began to feel much better and was able to finish my high school education. When I graduated, I assumed that I would get well because I was away from the social and academic pressures of school. I guess I still wasn't willing to admit that my depression wasn't circumstantial. I didn't want to believe that there was something wrong with me. I preferred to blame my environment for causing my problems. Being strong willed and stubborn, I decided to go off my medication. My first term at college was miserable, and I had my worst bout of depression yet. Besides the emotional strain, I wasn't able to eat or sleep at all, and I had a lot of physical pain as well. I felt like I had a huge lump in my chest that I couldn't get rid of. It was almost impossible to swallow, and there was nothing I could do about it.

When I was studying, I was so tense that I felt like screaming or kicking something really hard. I felt as if my muscles were going to jump out of my skin. During my daily routine of academics and athletics, I had to fit in about two hours of total dysfunction. I would sit in the library and study for a while and then I would cry. I would call my mother and cry over the phone, or go for a walk and cry. I finally broke down and told my roommates what was happening with me to my surprise they were very understanding. My roommate suggested I try marijuana in a herbal tea or smoke it in a pipe. She said she would get some from her boyfriend and give it to me to try. A few days later I tried the marijuana. I smoked some and right away I felt the difference. I stopped crying and I could eat and sleep again. I went back on my medications as well and my roommates boyfriend got me the medical marijuana, when I needed it.

Depression is not a rational thing. Most people don't understand it, which is why I don't tell too many of my friends about my illness. When I was finally diagnosed with major depression, I was relieved that there was a reason for my emotional distress. Once I realized that my depression was not something that I was responsible for, and once I understood that I had a chemical imbalance in my brain, everything began to improve. When I was able to say, "this illness is not caused by something I did wrong, and it's not my fault," I felt a certain freedom. It took me awhile to come to grips with the realization that my illness is something I will have to cope with for the rest of my life. Luckily, I have some wonderful women friends who have been invaluable to me. Another important source of support for me was my cats, and they still are. This may sound ridiculous, but they have always been a security blanket for me. When I was younger and the cats were close to my size and weight, I would carry them around. When I would get upset I would grab a cat and cry into its neck. Even now, during my school vacations, I'm drawn back home because that's where my animals are. I need to spend a certain amount of time with them. Even when I was in crisis I took the initiative and did everything I knew to do. The medical marijuana changed my life. I can take action on my behalf but it's also allowed me to make good decisions for myself. I consider myself a perfectionist, but being on antidepressants and medical marijuana I have the ability to be more evenly balanced. Since I've gotten so much better my life has also changed for the better. I have fewer worries now that I know I have a handle on my illness. I have much more freedom because I have a better idea of I need to do. I won't be as blindsided as I was early on when I didn't have a clue what was happening. I tried my best, It's like everything in life. You adjust, you learn to deal with things and you work around them. We have a real strong sense of family. If anything we're probably all closer because of what we've gone through.

We've all worked together with a common goal. In families like ours, one of two things usually happens, a pulling apart, or a pulling closer together. We've a much closer, stronger family because of my mental illness. We've a very religious family, and that has a lot to do with holding us together. Our faith gives us our values, it gives us our principles, and it gives us our direction. The little things that everyone for granted are things I just can't do. I know that people often stare at me. I'm not oblivious to what goes on. At first, I was embarrassed about my illness. On TV, if someone goes to see a psychiatrist, other folks say to them "Oh, you're a mental patient". Although sometimes it's funny on TV, it makes people feel ashamed to say, "I have to go see a psychiatrist. I really don't know how to describe my depression, because each person has different symptoms. It's hard for everyone who has it. It's hard and it's scary. It's definitely a lot of work, and it's not something fun to have. It's not something you're pretend to have. No one would want to live like this. It's unbelievable how much love and support there is in this family, and that helps a lot. Maybe some families don't have that love. I stay on top of my medications and medical marijuana every day and I'm completely involved in the process of getting well. If I'm having a stressful day, I'll adjust my dosage myself. My doctor supports me in this. It's empowering to take control over my illness and not let it control me. I believe that you get from life what you put into it. I'm learning to stop complaining about my problems, and instead, use that negative energy to do something about them in a positive way. It's up to me to make my life the way I want it to be. It's my responsibility. I never realized this before I got sick, but after getting better it became clear that I was in control of my life. I am in control more and more everyday and gaining more confidence in myself. My self esteem has improved and I no longer feel that I need to identify myself as having depression. I'm myself first. I feel like I got a second chance and I want to give back to the mental health community. I've been on the board of the County Alliance for the mentally ill for the past two years. I want to be an advocate for those mentally ill people who don't have the ability to speak for themselves. I've been there myself and now I want to help others. I consider the mentally ill, my people to. Anonymous

I came from skid row all the way up to where I'm at today. When I first went to a mental health clinic about fifteen years ago . I had no place to live. I had been wandering in the streets for years with hardly any money coming in. Something I worked very hard to make happen. I'm proud that I finally found a place of my own that I can call home. I'm proud that I have a permanent address. It's not the best looking apartment in the world but it's home. In the past, I had to hustle. Now I don't have to worry about where I'm going to shower, make dinner, or where I'm going to lay my head down at night. Things are better for me now, but I've had a lot of problems since I was a young kid. In elementary school, I was violent. The kids used to tease me because I was slow, and I would beat them up. Later on, I got into trouble for fighting in high school. I started seeing psychiatrists, but they never could pinpoint why I was so aggressive. I was also very depressed. The doctors thought that it was just an anger thing. I was a mediocre student in high school. I was in special education classes because I had some kind of disability as far as learning goes. It wasn't until about six months before my graduation that I got serious. I graduation by the skin of my teeth. I was the only one in my family who had ever finished high school. My mother was very proud to see one of her kids do good. Growing up there was only my mother, my younger sister, and me in my family. My dad was never around when he had to deliver child support or when he wanted to see us. One time he asked me, "what do you want from me"? I said "what I want is a father, not a drinking buddy who comes to see me once a month". I wanted a dad to throw a football around with and to go with to a ballgame. Stuff like that. A normal childhood. It never happened, so I depended on other people to be like a father to me. As I got older, my dad had kids with another woman, and didn't want to see him anymore. One day my half brother called me and told me that my father had died. I didn't shed a tear, I didn't do anything. I showed up for the funeral because I wanted to make sure my dad was dead. I began to get involved with a lot of things that I shouldn't have, like gangs and drugs. My mother and I drifted apart, but a year before she died, she and I became real close again. I depended a lot on my mother. When she died in January 1986, everything changed. I was just out of high school, and I didn't really know how to survive. Folks in my family took in my sister, I was left on my own and I did what I had to do to get by. I got depressed and I ran away. I didn't see my sister for maybe three of four years. I was just out wandering on the streets, sleeping on park benches in churches, in parking lots, and any where I knew I would be safe. There were times that it got real cold and rainy. There were a lot of police stations downtown near skid row, and they gave out vouchers for a local hotel. The police knew me well. I was no trouble maker so sometimes they'd even let me sleep in one of the empty jail cells. That way, I could stay out of the rain and have breakfast in the morning. Somehow I managed to go to school, even though I was homeless. I got financial aid from the school by using the addresses of friends in my neighborhood. I had always loved to cook, so I took a culinary class. When I finished the course, I found a job, but I was still living from place to place.

Although things in my life seemed to be going a little better for me, my violence continued to get me into trouble. When I got my first job with the state, I worked in a program where you go out in emergencies, like flash floods to help people out. I beat up one of my coworkers for saying something rude to me, leaving him with a broken nose, a fractured arm and three missing teeth. I knew something was wrong with me, but nobody would tell me what was causing me to be so violent. With my friends who knew me well, I'm as gentle as a lamb. But piss me off and I'm a raging bull that's going to come after you. I had a seizure at work one day and ended up in the hospital. After they did a CT Scan, the doctors thought that I had a brain tumor. It turns out I had hydrocephalus, which is fluid backing up in my brain. The specialist who was in charge of the neuron-surgery department said to me "John, I could save your life by putting a shunt in your head, but your life. If you don't want me to save your life now, you'll die within the next six months". He explained that my brain was already at the point of blowing up. After a week of pain and agony, I decided to have the surgery. When I first found out about having Hydrocephalus, I was really depressed. They had me see one of the psychiatrists in the hospital, and he told me, "you have bipolar disorder". I said, " you're telling me that on top of all that I'm going through, I also have to deal with having a mental illness? But then he told me about what bipolar disorder was, and I felt at ease with the diagnosis. I knew that my behavior was kind of weird. I'd feel real depressed one day, and then the next day or so I would be real panicky and sometimes violent. One I understood what was wrong with me, I said, okay, what do I do now? The doctor gave me some meds and told me to go to a mental health clinic. I didn't show up at the mental health clinic for four years because I thought I don't need to do it. I was still living with my sister at the time. She noticed that I was mixing my meds with alcohol and stuff. There were times when I took too much medication on purpose, and I would get up in the middle of the night and crash. My sister had this glass table and I don't know exactly what happened, but she said that I fell on the table. The next morning, there were bruises all over my body. I became suicidal. Even after thirteen suicide attempts, I still wanted to die. I didn't know what my purpose in life was. As far as having a profession in cooking. I couldn't get a job in a restaurant because no one was going to hire somebody who had seizures. I felt like the work I loved had been taken away from me. Four years after my diagnosis, I finally went to a mental health clinic, where I met a social worker named Sally. She became my case manager. To this day, I think of her as a saint. I could always turn to Sally for encouragement. If I felt like I couldn't do something, she was there to tell me I could. Even though things were working out for me at the clinic, I was still getting violent. There was one client there who was taunting me and raising hell about stuff. One day, I grabbed him by the throat and I wouldn't let him go. All the staff came, but nobody could get me off him because I'm too big. By the time they finally pulled me away from the man he was blue in the face. They had to give him CPR. My sister knew everything that was going on with me. One day we had a long talk about my illness. She suggested I try some marijuana for a calming effect. She got me some and I tried it. It works for me. I'm less violent and have more self control. Medical marijuana plus my meds keep me in check and my mental illness under control.

It's more like the marijuana relaxes me so I don't get upset at things that normally would get me upset. I started to think differently and not let my emotions take over as I did in the past, which turned into a violet tirade at times. For me, marijuana is a medicine that helps me every day to deal with what life brings me. I now call it medical marijuana because it is medicine that works for me. Naturally I still get angry at some things but I can control it now. I also have become a better cook in the kitchen. I'm able to concentrate better on the different types of dishes that I am learning how to do. And the dishes that I know how to do are coming out better. Thanks to medical marijuana, I haven't attacked anyone in maybe a good four or five years now. That's a miracle! It's a long time for me because I have an urge to fight. Now with medical marijuana if you piss me off, I might cuss under my breath or cuss them out. But I've learned to control my temper. There was a time when a mental health group was trying to put up some new housing for the mentally ill in a neighborhood, but the neighbors didn't want it there. I went to a meeting but that didn't help. This attitude comes from the news papers and TV people have this negative view of the mentally ill. So they don't want to live near them. The rumors start with sparks and become like a wildfire running. I believe that needs to change. We're not these monsters that we've been made out to be. We are people too and we're productive members of our communities. We have a lot of great recovery stories. People with mental illness are a recovery stories. People with mental illness are a very proud type of people because we've had to work harder to improve our lives. We have to fight for whatever little piece of the pie that society is willing to give us. I don't know if the stigma of mental illness will be reduced during my generation, but I hope with the help of the young people who are being educated about it, there will be some kind of a breakthrough. I just want to get to see the stigma stop, hopefully it will. Now I am able to hold down a part time job as a short order cook. Of cause it's not like I'm working at a fancy restaurant but it gives me a little money and I'm doing something that I like to do. Being that I'm working part time that gives me free time to do whatever personal matters I have to do. My life is far from perfect and may never be but it's getting better and better every day. Anonymous

Testimonials

My husband, Bill and I have four sons, all of whom are grown. When we tell the story of our oldest son James, we say the real tragedy is that his story is not unique. James who is now forty-eight, has schizoaffective disorder. He has been sick ever since he was seventeen. As a child, James never acted out. He didn't fight or rebel in any way. He was very attached to his family, was active in Church activities, and received all kinds of academic honors. His life seemed to be going in all the right directions. When James went to college, his pattern became a bit rocky. He excelled in the courses he was interested in, but he didn't bother to go to many of his other classes. He just wouldn't show up for them. This was so unlike him that Bill and I thought it was very strange. James also wasn't returning his library books and he would get huge bills for his overdue books. There were all these subtle signs that there might be something wrong. James continued to have a rocky time of it after he left college. He lived nearby and worked in a publishing company doing research. He also opened an art gallery. He had unlimited energy. But then he lost his job, and the gallery fell apart financially. When James moved to Colorado, Bill and I began to get bizarre letters from him. These letters were filled with strange ideas. James would mention people who were beaming messages down to him, and tell us how he had just exorcised his dog. It was c all very odd. For the first time, I acknowledged to myself that he might be psychotic. James's girlfriend began to call us because she felt threatened by him. He blamed all his problems on his girlfriend. When his girlfriend decided to leave him, her father was so nervous about James that he took a security guard with him to pick up her things but there was still a confrontation between James and the guard.

Things got so bad for James that he was evicted from his apartment and ended up living in his car for a while. We persuaded him to come back home. We tried to get him to go see a therapist, but he refused. Bill and I and our three younger sons decided to see a psychiatrist to get some guidance. He was very helpful. He told us James might be mentally ill. James began to threaten us. When his behavior was considered dangerous by the legal system, he was hospitalized and diagnosed with bipolar disorder. This was the first real understanding of what was wrong with James. James wouldn't accept help of any kind, so the hospital instructed us to get a court order for treatment for him. We did so, and treatment was ordered. This was family intervention at work. The Lawyer assigned to our son James fought to protect James rights. Both James and his Lawyer threatened to sue the hospital, so the hospital released him without treatment. This simply confirmed James's belief that there was nothing wrong with him. James began to turn against us. As parents, we had to make the decision to go to court so that James would receive treatment. If James had been diagnosed with a life threatening medical condition and was resisting treatment or surgery for it, we would have done the same thing. The psychiatrist warned us that we might become the enemy in James's eyes.

He was right. We hoped that if James was required to take medications, he would get better and understand why we had taken this action. Unfortunately this didn't happen. After he left the hospital he lived on the streets and in the woods outside of town. He came to our house several times in the middle of the night and yelled and screamed obscenities. If his brothers were there, they would try to reason with him, but nothing worked. The neighbors would call the police out of sheer frustration. We finally got a restraining order to keep him at least one hundred feet from our home because the police told us that it was the best thing for us to do. There were times when the police would take James to the State Hospital, but he would be out again in a matter of hours. It was a revolving door kind of thing. We were all incredibly frustrated and frightened. One night, James broke into our house while Bill and I were asleep. He beat us badly and almost killed me. We had a large house and the neighbors couldn't hear us calling for help. Fortunately, our son Robert and his wife were living with us at the time the Department of Mental Health got involved in his case and managed to arrange for James to be involuntarily committed to a State Hospital for an evaluation after he was released from jail.   James was found to be mentally ill and a danger to others. The Department of Mental Health attempted to get a court order to keep him in the hospital for at least six months. The lawyers were assigned to him case, but James just kept firing them. The judge ordered James to be brought into the court room with his hands and feet shacked. There was an armed guard watching him at all times. James was allowed to act as his own lawyer. He claimed that Bill wasn't his father. I can't describe how awful it was. The judge would allow no medical or police records into evidence. It was as if we were in a first degree murder situation instead of what was simply a civil hearing to determine whether the court could mandate treatment for our son. The judge released him. James was free to go. He simply disappeared.

For five long years we had no idea where James was, or if he was dead or alive. The homeless and missing persons network searched for him to no avail. We hired a private investigator and he promised us that he would find our son James and he did. James was in jail. Without provocation, he had seriously assaulted another man who had befriended him.

In his delusional state of mind James believed that the man had been stalking him. James was evaluated and diagnosed with paranoid schizophrenia, but he was still found competent to stand trial. There were two trials. He refused to allow a plea of mental and he fired his lawyer, although the district attorney and the defense lawyers and judge were very kind and thoroughly understood that James was mentally ill, and they had to comply with the law. The trial resulted in a hung jury.

Bill and I went for the second trial, but James did not speak to us. During the proceedings he was allowed to defend himself. James's strange behavior and speech showed his paranoia, but the judge remained patient. This time, the jury found him guilty and James was sentenced to two years in prison. In prison, James refused treatment and it was obvious to the prison authorities that James has a mental problem and needs treatment. As the time came close to his release date, the mental health staff arranged for a civil commitment hearing. At that hearing, the judge mandated treatment for James in a State Hospital in Virginia. This was the first time that he ever received medication. Steady progress was reported to us. After six months James was transferred to another State Hospital. After a few more months he was released. The court ordered mandatory outpatient treatment for him, and a community based mental health team helped him find housing and work provided his medication. Unfortunately James still refused to be in contact with his family or friends. My husband Bill noticed the change right away this was the first time he was given medication and it changed his life. He also met a girl who he told everything about his illness. She seemed to really care for James and understood his illness and needs. Rachael was always there for James so the family really appreciate her for James. But what they didn't know was Rachael had agoraphobia. She told James and he had no problem with it. She told James about medical marijuana because it helped her so much along with her meds. She wanted him to try it. He was reluctant at first but he tried it. After a couple of puffs from a pipe and he felt instant relief and relaxation. So James began to take medical marijuana and his prescribed medicine to maintain himself. Bill and I are angry on behalf of our son and thousands like him who have suffered needlessly for years when court mandated treatment could have relieved the terrible symptoms of their mental illnesses.

When James assaulted us, there was so much media attention that we had no choice but to speak out. We felt we should try to make it understandable to the public. As a result, a lot of people have contacted us and have told us this has happened in our family to. Not only did they feel the stigma of mental illnesses but they also felt tremendous shame around the issue of violence. James was accepted at Yale, but when the college was informed by his high school, he was rejected, but he did get accepted at the University of Main. By his second year he was doing great and well on his way to a bright future as long as he remembered to take his meds along with medical marijuana. He graduated from the university and shortly after he married Rachael. He got a good job as an accountant and he and Rachael were expecting their first child in the Spring. Rachael and I want to make sure that people who are mentally ill will be helped by early intervention if they can't help themselves. When you've been to hell and back, what else can life do to you? Curiously enough, it gives you a certain freedom. At least, I think that's been true for us.

One thing I really regret is not keeping a journal over the years. So much has happened to our family that it's hard to keep track of it all. Both my husband George and my daughter Anna are mentally ill. George has been hospitalized four times, always on licked units. Anna has been in and out of hospitals ten times. George and I first noticed there was something wrong with Anna when she was in the second grade. She couldn't sleep alone in the dark, and she had other symptoms as well. She burned herself once and didn't react to the pain. She didn't cry. We brought her to see a therapist, who treated her for several years. When Anna's symptoms improved the therapist released her from treatment, however she told us our daughter might not make it through her adolescence without additional help. She was right. Where Anna went to high school her entire world fell apart. She began to hear voices, and she even made a suicide attempt. She had been a straight "A" student, but she ended up missing so much school that she had to drop out. But she went back the following year and graduated. I don't know how she did it. Anna got

97

very sick again in her twenties when she working at a hospital as a nursing assistant. George had two hospitalizations for manic depression in the summer of 1975, and two more in the winter of 1988. He was first hospitalized when our children were the ages of eight, ten and twelve. His mother was babysitting for us, and she called me and told me to come from work. There was something wrong with George. George had suddenly worked out work. We had to call the ambulance to take him to the State Hospital. He spent a month there, and after he was released, George tried going back to work. He ended up in the psych ward of the local hospital for another thirteen months. George has been seeing a therapist for years now. He's always known when he needs help. And he always seeks it. On the other hand, Anna took a long time to accept her mental illness. She resisted taking medication. She didn't want to go to her day treatment program. She fought everything! When Anna was in her twenties and going downhill, George and I went together to see a therapist who recommended a support group for families. It's been immensely helpful for us. When Anna was very sick, George wanted to help her he realized that he couldn't do that much for her, he thought maybe he could help someone else. Now he puts in forty-five hours a week as a relief worker at a group home for elderly men who cannot live alone, and at a shelter for homeless people who have been diagnosed with mental illness. He also works at a group home for women. I have never kept George's illness a secret from my family down south. I told them about his diagnosis when he first got sick. We've also visited family members when Anna wasn't well. Although there are some members of the family who find it difficult to talk about mental illness, They've all been supportive. Everyone has to deal with something. Sometimes you wonder whether you're going to make it or not, so you do what you have to do to get through a difficult time. When you love someone who is mentally ill and they're doing well, you're really happy about it.

Mental illness really hit my family hard. My sister was over fifty the first time she was hospitalized for manic depression. My brother was thirty six when he twenties, but she was already in therapy by the time she was in the second grade. I spent my twentieth birthday in a mental hospital. I had walked out of work in the middle of the day without telling anybody. On the way home, I stopped at a clinic to get some help. At that time, when there was no crisis intervention services in our town, so the clinic staff told me to try to hold out until Monday, when I already had an appointment with a counselor. I didn't make it until Monday. By Monday night, I was strapped to a bed in the State Hospital. I spent a month in the hospital. I was released in time for the fourth of July, but the next week I had to be readmitted to the local psych ward, where I spent another three months before my insurance ran out. I returned to work, but hit a seasonal layoff a few weeks later. I job hunted and collected unemployment for the next fourteen months, until the state rehabilitation department found me a job. I stayed at the job for the next sixteen years. In late December 1990, I became very stressed out, worrying about the future of me job and watching my father go through the same thing. Three months after Anna's first hospitalization, I knew that I was headed for trouble again, so I admitted myself to the hospital for the first time in sixteen years. The doctors didn't think much was wrong with me, and they released me after six days without monitoring the medication they had prescribed. I tried to go back to work just two days later. I knew I was still a little wired, bit I thought I had it under control. I didn't. My boss had to call my mother to come get me. A day later, I was back in the hospital for another ten days, and this time, I was put in restraints. I had a bout of insomnia, and I went ninety-five hours with only four hours of sleep. But there was a young girl in the hospital who hadn't slept in fourteen days.

They ended up sending her for electroshock treatment. At one point, I attempted to help her escape from the hospital. I never found out what happened to her after that. After I got out of the hospital the second time the State Rehabilitation office got me another job. I never attempted to hide my background at work it just so happens that's how I got the job. Only one person at work has ever asked me about my illness. I'd sit in the cafeteria with him and talk about my situation. I confided in him, he seemed to really care. In our conversation he made me aware of medical marijuana and what it would do. After work we went to his house and he helped me smoke it. If only I knew about this before along with my medication I would never had all the problems. I have through the years. It's a tough decision whether to tell a prospective employer that you are mentally ill. If the Americans with disabilities act, but if you do tell them, they can find ways to get around the disabilities act, and they may get rid of you anyway.

With the help of medical marijuana I've gotten so much better, I've been doing a lot of public speaking about mental illness. People often wonder how I can go up in front of groups like the Rotary Club and bare my soul. I've been lucky. My family has been very understanding and fortunately my parents are still together. Many marriages break up when someone in the family has a mental illness. Everyone has their breaking point, and some people can take more than others can. Because of deinstitutionalization, there are more mentally ill people in jail at any given time than there are in all the psychiatric hospitals put together. People were taking out of the state hospitals and put out on the street before support systems for them were available in their communities. Sixty percent of the people who were released from our local state hospital went off their medications within three months. Many of them ended up in jail or on the streets. I helped lead a forty week training session with a local police department. I told them that the mentally ill people they deal with are usually off their meds or refuse to take any. I want the police to know that for every mentally ill person they have to deal with, there are doctors and lawyers and school teachers and college presidents and people like me who are mentally ill and are doing very well. I still don't have a whole lot of self confidence, and I'm still introverted and bashful about approaching people. I there are lots of people who are better at interacting with other people than I am. I still worry that I'm going to do something wrong, but all in all, it's been very satisfying to help others. I'm going to graduate from a state college with a bachelor's degree in sociology in the spring I'm on disability and that's difficult for me. I want to be able to get a job that I can stick with, to stay out of the hospital, to stay on my meds and medical marijuana and to do what I have to do. I haven't been hospitalized for over four years and now I'm engaged to a man I met while we were both patients during my last hospitalization. I'm doing so well now, I just count my blessings.

When my son, Ted was diagnosed with paranoid schizophrenia, it hit my wife Sophia, and me very hard. We didn't even know exactly what it meant. Six months later, our son was dead. Everything happened so fast. We never had time to adjust to his illness and Ted didn't have the time to adjust to it either. My wife and I didn't know how severely sick Ted had been until his death. We should have recognized the early warning signs of mental illness years ago, but unfortunately, you often learn about these kinds of things after the fact. If only you could stop somebody before they make a decision to commit suicide. Our son never had an opportunity to become the person he wanted to be. The hardest thing my wife and I ever had to do was write Ted a letter and tell him he had to leave our home unless he began to participate fully in his own care. He was almost twenty-two years old and he was still living up in his bedroom. When Ted moved out of our house and got his own place, he went into a crisis. That's how we were able to get him to go to the hospital. When Ted was hospitalized, he was put on many different medications in an effect to find the right one. He suffered from their side effects. His hands would tremble, and he would drool. Although Ted seemed to be pretty well stabilized when he left the hospital, he still took his own life. He never even had enough time to get on the right medication. Ted was using medical marijuana and it helped him a lot but he still needed the right medication, the marijuana alone just wasn't enough, but it helped tremendously with Ted's side effects from the med's he was being given. We felt sure the medical marijuana and medications would help him a lot, but he didn't get that chance. We didn't mind him smoking marijuana because we could see how it made him feel, what a difference if only he had the right meds we feel he would be alive today. Ted ever wanted to be a burden to anybody. He told us many times not to worry about him. When he was discharged from the hospital, the staff recommended that he become independent as quickly as he could and provide for himself. They wanted him to go back to his own apartment and support himself without our help. If we had to do it all over again, we wouldn't do it the same way. We wouldn't have had Ted go back out on his own so soon because now we know that he just wasn't capable of living independently.

We understand now that the most critical time for people who are suicidal is when they are thinking clearly. They see their stretching out before them and they think, "what kind of a future do I really have"? They make a assessment of what their future holds. I think that's what Ted was struggling with. He was thinking clearly at the time of his suicide. He just didn't like his options. Ted committed suicide when he was twenty-two. My wife and I have often been asked. " who do you blame for Ted's death"? The only person we can blame is Ted. He made a terrible choice, I think he just got tired of struggling with his illness. Ted was a joyous happy child, when he was about fourteen, we saw a change in him. He got very sad and quiet and didn't seem happy. We assumed this was because his best friend had leukemia and was at deaths door. His friend recovered, but Ted didn't. He was in a very deep depression. We took him to a doctor, who confirmed that he was suffering from a form of "teenage depression". We thought that when he passed through his teenage years, his depression would go away. We never considered that he might be mentally ill. We thought that when he passed through his teenage years, his depression would go away. Ted was very talented musically. When he was seventeen, he started to play the guitar and write music. He also took piano lessons. He played beautiful, we brought him an electric piano. Soon after that, however we started to see a disturbing pattern in Ted's behavior. Ted never stuck with anything, his interest only lasted for short periods of time. He didn't even continue his piano playing. Ted began to withdraw, and he got quieter and quieter. When Ted was seventeen he decided he wanted to drop out of high school. After he dropped out Ted wanted to go to Ohio with some of his older friends. We told him he had to save enough money to pay for your transportation to get there and pay for two months rent for an apartment. To our dismay he sold his guitars, his valuable books, and his records. In two weeks Ted had everything together and he left for Ohio. Ted was in Ohio for less than a year. When we spoke to him on the phone, we realized that he wasn't well. He seemed fearful of so many things. Ted came back home to live with us because he felt much safer there. Ted wasn't able to hold a job. The people he worked for at McDonalds all liked him, but he felt like he never did good enough job. Ted's last job was in the pressman at a local newspaper. He would often have conversations with himself. Ted became increasingly frightened of so many things.

He was afraid of his food, afraid that somebody would come through the TV set and get him, afraid that somebody was in his closet or under his bed. During this, Ted began to do all kinds of artwork. He was a gifted artist even though he'd never taken any art lessons. Ted never appreciated the beauty and talent of his work. Ted was a big reader. He would read everything from books on Zen Buddhism to comic books and everything in between. There were many nights when my husband and I would just hold onto each other and not say a word because being so afraid for our son. Ted was our only child, and as parents, we are supposed to make our children better. We couldn't do that. I was naïve enough to believe that my love heals everything, but it really doesn't. It gets you through things, but it can't make anybody better. Ted's depression was hard for everyone in the family but I think my husband and I were the only ones who could understand what he was going through. We didn't really understand it at all. I'm not sure anyone can understand mental illness unless they experience it themselves. We even went into counseling together because we felt we had to go somewhere to learn to become better parents in order to become stronger for Ted and to understand him as much as we possibly could. When Ted was twenty-one we took him to a hospital. He told us he needed to rest because his mind was so tired. Ted seemed to begin to understand that he had a mental illness. Ted often worried about the stigma of mental illness and about how he was being perceived by others. People often spoke to him as if he were either retarded or deaf. Ted wanted his father to get him out of the hospital but that wasn't going to happen until Ted was feeling and doing better. But I soon realized he didn't mean "out" of the hospital. He meant out of this life. The intensity of his words was reflected in his eyes. There was no doubt in my mind that Ted wanted to end his life. In retrospect, I wish I had picked up on some of the warning signs that Ted might be close to taking his life. Ted's father and I were planning to go to

Maine on the Friday before Father's Day and we were to come on that Sunday, we found Ted. He had taken his life., it was Father's Day. After Ted's death, I felt like a ship tossed and tumbled all about. My husband and I sometimes say to each other, We never be happy again. But then we realized it's a day to day thing. It's hard to understand mental illness unless you know someone who experience it. You think of the mentally ill as "those people", like the ones who talk to themselves on the street corner in the rain. You think, "Oh those poor people!" You don't ever think of someone like Ted who could carry on a conversation, move into his own apartment and act just like anybody else, as a person who could take his own life. I don't think anybody realized just how sick he was. No matter what, if you know someone who is mentally ill, don't ever give up hope. There's always some hope. Try to be with that person and teach them about the wonderful things that can come out of life. Tell them about the good things they can do and how many people they can help. I would like to tell people that it's not their fault if they have a mental illness, and that it's not s big deal if they do. If they are mentally ill, it doesn't mean that they're any less of a person. Anybody can get a mental illness. Anybody.

TESTIMONIAL

On the day my husband and I moved into our beautiful, brand new home, I remember thinking I had everything I'd ever dreamed of. At thirty-eight, I was happily married to my college boyfriend we had two healthy sons, and I loved my work as a clinical social worker in a hospital. In retrospect, this period in my life was just the calm before the storm. There were problems on the horizon. My father had suffered a stroke and was slowly dying. My mother, who was an invalid needed to go into a nursing home since my dad could no longer take care of her. I was most troubled, however, by the discovery that my husband's pacemaker had a defective part that could crack and kill him instantly. During the month we had to wait before it could be removed. I couldn't sleep more than four hours a night. I would lie awake just watching him breathe. With so much stress in my life, I started to fall apart emotionally. I began to have psychotic thoughts. I became convinced that my conversations were being taped, and that my office was bugged. Their ideas just came into my head. My thoughts seemed so real. One day, I told a coworker that we were all under surveillance at the office. She immediately informed my supervisor, who called my husband to tell him that I wasn't acting like myself. When Greg came to pick me up at work, I insisted there was nothing wrong with me, and that it was simply a misunderstanding. I didn't hear voices or anything, but I thought I was communicating with something that was tapping coded messages into my ears. It was crazy stuff. I talked too fast, I laughed too much, and said inappropriate things. I even told a few doctors at work to stop cheating on their wives. I'm usually the most conservative, rule- following, least troublemaking person anyone could ever meet, but one day I was walking down the hallway at work and I had this thought that pulling the fire alarm would be a neat thing to do. Fortunately, I didn't set it off, but I almost did. I could have done anything. I felt like I could go into the operating room at the hospital where I worked and do surgery on patients. Luckily, I didn't attempt to do that, either. I began to have even more delusions. At one point, I thought Greg was going to poison the children and me, and I also believed that the FBI wanted me to work on a top secret project. Greg was so worried about me that one day, when I was about to take a bath Greg told me to leave the door unlocked he was afraid I could drown myself. He pleaded with me to see a doctor, but I insisted that I was fine and had everything under control. I became convinced my husband was planning to sabotage my grandiose plans to work for the FBI. I hired a lawyer and filed for divorce. A few weeks later, I moved into a small apartment near our house. Even-though I was still trying to care for the boys, I wasn't capable of it. I asked Greg to keep them. I told my sons that I loved them very much but that I had to leave them with their dad for a while. Even though I was so sick and totally psychotic, I still had sound maternal instincts. I was trying to protect my babies because I knew they would be safer with Greg. Giving our kids to him was the most painful thing I've ever done. When I'd go visit them, they'd cry when I left to go back to my apartment. It just broke my heart. This was the loneliest time of my life. I felt absolutely worthless and hopeless. A few weeks after moving into my apartment, my dad died. I went to his funeral in Ohio and gave the eulogy even though I was completely psychotic at the time.

I thought I was being taped, and I was convinced that the funeral director was in love with me. In our family, I've always been seen as someone in control of my life. My relatives didn't know what to make of my unusual behavior. They assumed it was caused by the street of losing my father. When I returned home, I started giving away my furniture and clothing to strangers. I would knock at people's doors and leave stuff for them. I gave away a nice fur coat and my beautiful lace wedding dress and I sold my wedding ring for dirt. One night I packed up my sets of dishware and silverware and left them on a doorstep in a poor section of town. I even through away precious family photos. By then, Greg had hired detectives to follow me because he suspected was having an affair. Even though he believed I would never do something like that, he needed a reason to explain my behavior. He was in denial about the reality of my illness. I would sometimes lie on the floor of my apartment catatonic, when a neighbor came in and found me like this, she offered to get me some supper, but I couldn't even get up to eat. I was that depressed, that sick. I alienated every relationship I had. Greg and I were fighting all the time. My friends and family had given up on me because I was so obnoxious. I wasn't even able to be a good mother. My sister has schizophrenia and I began to worry that I would end up like her. I felt like some kind of leper. I went to a doctor who confirmed my diagnosis and gave me medication, around this same time a coworker told me about medical marijuana and how much it helped her and that I should try it. She brought me so me the next day. The marijuana along with my medication saved my life. What a difference! I slept eight hours straight for the first time in four months. It was a miracle. Then I was also given an antidepressant which helped stop my compulsive worrying. Thanks to the medical marijuana I felt sane again. Once I could think clearly, I was able to straighten out my life. I salvaged my marriage and I tried to be the best mom I could be. It was difficult, but I went back to work and faced all the people who had seen me behaving so erratically. I'm a social worker, and I think I'm more helpful now to folks than before I got sick. I realize that patients are afraid and I try to comfort them, to reassure them. I've learned from my own experience to be even more compassionate than I was before. I decided to share my experience so I could show people that there is hope for a happy life despite having a mental illness. My story was in a well known magazine and I've also written a book, been on TV and in the news paper. Even the most hopeless of situations can be turned around, for me it was the marijuana medication and therapy. The stigma against mental illness is definitely out there. I think one of the reasons why so many people have such a hard time with mental illness is that they worry it could happen to them or to someone they love. Mental illness can happen to anyone. If it does, you need to cope with it and not put your head in the sand. You need to deal with it and make the best of it. You don't need to be afraid of it. It's not a death sentence.

Stacy A. FAMILY'S HISTORY OF MENTAL ILLNESSES

My name is Stacy A.,. There is a history of mental illness in my family, which began with my grandfather. He had manic-depression and he committed suicide by jumping out of a fourteen story building in the 1930's. My father had manic-depression, too. He was a colonel in the marine corps., and his illness hit him during his thirtieth year in the military. He was forced to resign because he couldn't do his job properly. My father's brother, a priest, developed depression when I was seventeen, but I didn't know I was suffering from a mental illness. I was a cheerleader and I remember going to a football game and telling my boyfriend that I couldn't understand why I felt so sad. It was hard to go out on the field and pretend to be happy. I couldn't stay focused during my senior year of high school. I was working toward a 4.0. average because I wanted to go to a good college, but it became extremely difficult to hang on. Somehow, I was able to get through that year with an "A" average, and I was offered four scholarships to different colleges. I went to an Ivy League college, but I struggled emotionally and academically. I was able to finish up my freshman year in college, but the week before I went back to school for my sophomore year, my father had the first of many manic-depressive episodes and attempted suicide. This left me shaken, scared, and even more depressed. I tried to keep up with my studies, but I was simply not able to continue. I had no idea what was going on with me, no idea that I was also suffering from a mental illness. I know I had to take time off from school to try to cope with my father's illness and its effect on our family. I also need time to deal with my own mental and emotional struggles. I was filled with intense anguish when I realized that I couldn't keep up with my academic demands. I had to drop out of college and give up all my scholarships and grants. I clung to a normal life to the best of my ability, and two years later I went back to college. My father's worsening illness and my own undiagnosed depression affected my concentration, my memory, my ability to problem solve, and my ability to handle stress. I was unable to complete the semester, so I decided to drop out of college again. I finally gave up on school altogether. I got married and had two children, Jason and Bobby. After the birth of Bobby in 1984, I started having severe problems with depression again. That year, my father made his tenth attempt at suicide, and this time he succeeded. Soon after that, I was diagnosed with major depression and started on numerous drug trials. My emotional pain continued to worsen because the medications never completely stabilized me, not until I discovered medical marijuana, which made me feel like a new person. But without the marijuana I began to have severe side effects. When Bobby was seven, he also was diagnosed with depression and was treated successfully with antidepressants. My husband wasn't working at the time, so we no longer were able to pay for medical insurance. I couldn't continue to get the kind of high quality psychiatric help that Bobby needed, because I just couldn't afford it. It took heaven and earth to find a good psychiatrist who would accept state health insurance.

When Bobby was thirteen, we finally found a psychiatrist who worked with poor people. It soon became obvious to me that she didn't give a damn about any of the children she was treating. She told me "Bobby's not depressed. He doesn't need to be on antidepressants anymore". She took him off all his medication even though he had attempted suicide the year before she saw him in treatment. How much more evidence did she need that Bobby was depressed? Three weeks after he stopped taking his medications,

Bobby committed suicide. He hung himself in the backyard of my mom's house. I have a lot of anger and resentment about this. I wonder why I couldn't get decent psychiatric help for my son. It could have saved his life. He was a good, kind intelligent, wonderful human being. His life was worth saving. Before Bobby died, I had gone off my meds because none of them were working except the medical marijuana. After he died, I was hospitalized immediately, and then entered various treatment facilities to help me with my depression and grief. In 1995, I was in a residential treatment facility that encouraged its clients to return to school. I signed up for classes that fall, but the week they started was the one- year anniversary of Bobby's death. I was hospitalized again for six weeks and had sixteen electroshock sessions to treat my severe depression. I not only forgot who I was, but also where I was, where I lived, my enrollment at school, and even the fact that my son had died. As my memory slowly returned, I had to relive his death all over again. I was not fully functional or cognizant at that time. Depression is an oppressive darkness and gloom. No happiness. No spark for life. It is sitting in a corner unable to move. It felt like a physical weight prevented me from being able to do ordinary, everyday things, like brushing my teeth or organizing my medications. The simplest aspects of living that most people take for granted, like deciding what shirt to wear, became impossible for me. I wasn't capable of cleaning my house, taking a slower, taking care of myself at all. I had absolutely no concentration. I had difficulty speaking and talking. I couldn't formulate sentences. I stuttered, I isolated myself, staying in my room for days at a time, and didn't go out or talk to anyone. I was angry a lot of the time. I felt very much alone, very guilty, and very ashamed of my mental illness. I blamed my illness for the death of my son because he didn't receive the protection, love, and support that he needed at the most critical time in his life.

This guilt is still difficult to bear. I spent many years on a quest to find a good doctor for myself. At his suggestion, I joined an intensive partial hospitalization program for four hours a day. My family members felt less responsible for me because they knew that professionals were overseeing the physical, emotional, and mental aspects of my life. My family was relieved not to have to play so many different roles in my life, which they'd never really been trained to handle in the first place. A turning point in my recovery came when I turned over the decision- making about my illness to professionals. I finally acknowledged that, not unlike an alcoholic, I wasn't in control of my illness and that I needed to give other people control over my treatment in order to get better. When I met my current psychiatrist, I began to do this, but I didn't do it all at once. It was a gradual process of letting go. I slowly learned to let the clinic staff help make decisions for me. It was very difficult to accept their input at first, but I soon saw that their advice helped me pull my life back together again. It took me a year to stabilize. I am currently on fourteen different medications and in intensive therapy. My psychiatrist has supported my intention to return to school, provided I only take six units a semester. I can't go back to school until I get some financial aid, and so far, I haven't received any. I've just written a letter to the financial aid office explaining my mental health history in the hope that they will reconsider my request for help. Thank goodness for medical marijuana,. I've become stable, I am a more loving, calm and logical person. I'm not as reactionary as I used to be. In the past, I would overreact to certain situations in our family. It was a hardship for my children because I would respond so inappropriately. At the time, I was angry, irritable, and not functioning most of the time. But, thank God, I kept looking for help. I have to protect my stability, and my family helps me do that by reducing my stress, by not letting me take on too much, and by keeping my life balanced physically, mentally, emotionally, and spiritually. My family who live in another city, all assist me in maintaining that balance. I constantly turn to m them with help making decisions.

Congenital Anomalies

Testimonials - Congenital Scoliosis and Inherited Genetic Trait

Sandy C has SCOLIOSIS CONGENITAL

Sandy C. was born with Scoliosis Congenital (curvature of the spine) that did not affect her until the age of 32 years old. Sandy was a Postal worker that sorted mail to be transferred to other States for local delivery. This job is a physical labor job where a person has to lift heavy mail bags and boxes. One day while Sandy was working she lifted several heavy mail bags and felt a slight pain in the lower part of her back. At first she thought it was a little strain but the next morning she felt great pain in her back, and decided to take the day off from work and rest her body for a day. The next morning she felt the same great pain in her back, so she called in sick and went to her doctor. The doctor said that she had a pinched nerve that was caused by a combination of over straining and the curvature of her spine.

The doctor referred her to a specialist in that field and he told her that she might have to have back surgery to try to correct the problem. He also told her that there was a chance that she might have nerve damage after the surgery and it might affect her motion. She asked the doctor, "What do you mean, might affect motion?" He told her that there is a possibility that she might lose the motion in one of her legs or both of her legs. She said, you mean I might not be able to walk again after surgery? The doctor said, yes, it's possible. The doctor said, don't think about it now, there might be other alternatives that can be utilized. The doctor saw the fear in Sandy's eyes when he told her that she might not walk again after the surgery. So he told her that there might be other alternatives but in his mind surgery was the only cure. Sandy went home to think about it, and in the mean while she would go out on disability from the Post Office. Sandy went to another doctor and he said that it is possible that she would not need surgery. She would have to see several doctors that specialize in spinal treatment and back treatment. She would have to change her eating habits and the types of food she was used to eating, being that she was over weight for her height. Sandy began to eat more nutritional foods and began to go to health food stores and herbal stores. She started to learn about herbal medications for pain and to improve health. She was making great progress but still having pain and discomfort. Sandy took pain killers but she felt the pain killers were too strong for just discomfort, so she would take a combination of vitamins and herbal medication that included marijuana for discomfort. Sandy also stated that she stop taking sleeping pills to go to sleep and instead took marijuana as a sleep aid, that did not leave her groggy in the morning like sleeping pills did. There are some of the other vitamins and herbal medications that Sandy is taking. Multi-Vitamins and Minerals, Salmon Oil soft gel tablets, Iron pills, Devil's Claw, Asian Ginseng, Cod-liver Oil.

Fabona P suffers an INHERITED GENETIC TRAIT

Fabona P. is a middle aged man that suffers from a real genetic inherited trait in his families ancestral line. The trait affects the male decedents twice as much as the female decedents. This real genetic trait affects the males with amplification of one's senses to intolerable degrees. For example Fabona became very sensitive to sound, light, smells, and touch to his body. At the age of 35 the family trait began to affect him in noticeable ways. Fabona would say that even the slightest sound of a mouse inside of a wall would sound like an elephant marching inside of there. Fabona would wear dark glasses because the normal light would cause unbearable pain. The trait starts to progress at middle age and advance. This type of inherited mania has almost driven Fabona insane. But Fabona knew his family history with two servants. The family's wealth which was considerable would provide for his needs. He would have to take different medications to help him deal with his problems. He would only eat certain foods and drinks. With this type of illness the stress comes automatically every day. Fabona would have the servants to keep the window drapes drawn to keep out sun light and have them work quietly in the house to lower the noise of activity. He would not let the servants use certain cleaning fluids that would be intolerable to his sense of smell which was very acute. Some might think these are peculiarities of temperament but highly unlikely. This disorder goes back for many generations in Fabona's family history. He would take medical marijuana in hot tea and in ice tea to calm down his stress levels and relax his nerves. He would take other medications at different times. He also receives mental counseling to help him deal with this type of mania or phobia. The therapy are to increase self awareness, lean constructive ways of dealing with conflicts, establish a better sense of inner direction. When Fabona would leave the house he would wear dark glasses for the sun, ear plugs to keep out loud sounds and his body covered with soft cloth under his regular clothing. And of cause gloves for his hands with a sensitive touch. When other people would see him some would say that, he looks strange or weird. But he did not care what people said about him or what they thought about him or what he looked like. He only cared about surviving in the outside world until he went back home. Naturally he would limit his time in the outside world so that he could return to the safety and sanctuary of his home.

Fabona would spend most of his time painting pictures and reading books. Even though he could afford all the modern technology but he preferred to live the simple life. His paintings were very beautiful, some were landscape paintings, others were of things in general like people, animals, and beautiful places. He would always have to be aware of his condition and the environment that he was in like the boy in the bubble, protected from the ills of the outside world, protected in his own environment. He would take many different herbs and minerals with natural foods that were palatable to his taste. He was limited in the type of food products that he could eat. Being that his taste was amplified sweet things taste 10 times sweeter, and bitter n things tasted 10 times more bitter to him. He could not enjoy most of the food products that you and I have every day and take for granted. Fabona would say that medical marijuana in tea would relax him so he could concentrate on whatever he was doing at the time. He also would wear ear plugs and eye pads to bed before going to sleep. When he didn't do this he said, noises like rain drops outside his window sounded like the great rain. Which would keep him awake at night . And any amount of light would be bright enough to keep him awake. Fabona would have to continue these rituals for the rest of his life.

Due to having this illness all of life it had made him sensitive to details and a perfectionist in all aspects of his endeavors some people would think that Fabona was weird or strange or crazy. Probably in their minds he was but in reality he was not. There have been times in the past were he would even question his own sanity but realize that he would have to keep things in check and maintain his sanity.

it had came to pass that Fabona's paintings were noticed by the public and was selling very well. He was commissioned to paint a few peoples paintings which were beautiful when competed. As for people like Fabona their sense are more acute than the average person which makes them more sanative to detail in every situation. He being a privet solitude person did not like to associate with other people, only when necessary. Each one of his art projects took a long time from start to finish to make it as perfect as possible. Fabona is notorious for having to take medications including marijuana on a daily bases. Some people were lined up to commission him to do painting for them. When not painting for people he would live in seclusion away from people in his private world.

Digestive System, Nutrition and Metabolic Disorders

Bulimia Nervosa

BULIMIA NERVOSA

Bulimia nervosa which is an eating disorder that weight loss may occurs due to vomiting. It is estimated that 5% of all young women in college are affected by this disorder and is also seen in people whose occupation requires stringent weight control like models, actresses, jockeys, ballerinas.

Anorexia Nervosa

ANOREXIA NERVOSA

Anorexia Nervosa is the fear of gaining weight, so the patient does self imposed starvation because they think that they are too fat and have expressed dissatisfaction with aspects of their physical appearance. The most effective treatment for anorexia combines medical management, nutritional counseling, individual, group, or family psychotherapy. What should be addressed are the underlying problems of anxiety, guilt, low self esteem, depression and helplessness.

Anorexia nervosa is more common than people think. This disorder is a mental disorder due to emotional and inferior personality complex. The symptoms are the loss of appetite for food not caused by a disease. Loss of weight and appetite, more frequently occurs in girls and young women. Some people with this disorder believe that they are too fat and yet they appear to be under weight. Anorexia nervosa can occur in boys, men, and women. But is more common in young women may be because deep in subconscious there afraid of getting fat or old and feel this is the way to stay the same way. We cannot rule out depression as one of the factors involved. Pier presser could be another. Many people with this disorder will take medical marijuana as a appetite inducer as well as a antidepressant. Some people with this disorder will eat food just to satisfy their hunger and then soon after eating they will regurgitate the food out of there stomach. Reports have shown that in the United States anorexia nervosa affects 1 in 800 to 1 in 100 among adolescent females.

There are hundreds of different phobias that affect millions of people every day. These fears are from the mental psyche and can be treated in different ways. Phobias can be controlled with knowledge of the fear and learning why the person has the fear of a particular phobia and dealing with it. Medical marijuana has been used as a mild relaxer medication, to relax the phobic persons mind.

Everyone has had stress some time in their life. Some people hardly ever have stress and then some others have stress on a daily bases. There are different degrees of stress levels from low to high stress levels. The most common stress can be caused by ones job or life style or problem affecting ones physical, chemical changes. The term (stressed out) is frequently used which means at the maximum level. One does not think clearly and seems to loss energy and mental energy. 10, s of thousands will take medical marijuana to relieve their stressful feelings as well as relax.

Testimonials - Anorexia Nervosa

Connie E. suffers from ANOREXIA NERVOSA

Connie E. is suffering from Anorexia Nervosa and wasn't a where that she had the illness until her family notice a change in her appearance as of late. She is a 21 year old student of drama and the arts. All of Connie's family members are what's called heavy set people. Meaning a bit over weight except Connie which is about 100 lbs. Connie's mother loves to cook a lot of food every day but Connie is the only one that eats like a bird. Her mother always thinks that there is something wrong with Connie's appetite. Connie's brother and sister are also worried about Connie not eating. With Connie, she has a combination of problems that cause her not to eat properly. She had always resented that everyone in her family was heavy in body mass and didn't want that for herself. She had gotten in to a bad habit of not eating enough food for her height. She did not like purging food, instead she just would suppress her appetite and eat small amounts of food just to satisfy her hunger. In the past Connie would have the same meals like her brother and sister every day but as time moved on she began to dislike her family's appearance and didn't want that over weight appearance for herself. At times she was even ashamed of her family's appearance of looking over weight. Connie was so ashamed of her family that she would not invite her friends to come over her house. Connie's boyfriend Steve had no idea that Connie has a eating disorder until one day, when out on a date with Connie and all of the sudden Connie had fainted while walking down the street. Steve might have over reached when he called a ambulance to help Connie but it was a go thing he did. The Doctor at the hospital examined Connie and said that her body was very depleted and needed nutrients. The Doctor concluded by saying that Connie was a border line Anorexic and needed to eat more food. Steve was not surprised. This answered a lot of questions that Steve wonder about. Like why Connie would not eat all the food on her plate at dinner time or even have snack foods just to munch on. Connie also seem to have a lack of energy at times. She went to a Doctor that understands her disorder and prescribes medication and vitamins and a referral to a mental health Doctor for canceling. Connie seem to be in denial about her eating disorder and soon got over her in denial. Steve was very concerned about Connie's eating problem, and wanted to help her. But Steve knew that he would have to be careful on the way he would help her. Steve knows Connie's personality and she wouldn't like him constantly trying to get her to eat more. She would resent him sounding like the people in her family.

So he would try to get her to eat in such a way that it is all her idea to do so. Connie's mother started to make all of Connie's favorite foods at dinner time in the attempt to get her to eat more. Do you know the old saying "when it rains it poor's" well what Connie thought when she found out that she b was pregnant. Connie thought not only does she have to deal with her eating disorder but also a pregnancy. She realizing that she was only 21 years old and might not be ready to be a mother and yet she wanted a baby. First she would have to tell her parents and then tell Steve. Connie knew how her mother n would respond to the news of the pregnancy with over joy that she was going to be a Grandmother and a new life will; be born in the family. Whereas her farther would not be happy about Connie's pregnancy, so after a few days Connie told her mother first about the pregnancy. In doing so it left the job of telling Connie's farther, to her mother. After all the family members were told including Steve, it seem to be a joyous occasion for a short time. After a day or two the family members in clouding Steve began to talk amounts' them self's about Connie being Anorexic and pregnant and how it would affect the baby. It seem like the family members were conspiring to help Connie weather she wanted it or not. Naturally all the family's affords fail and only succeeded in driving Connie away from them. She felt that they were trying to control her life which made her angry. Connie was even more stressed but she knows that she has to eat nutritious foods during the pregnancy weather she is hungry or not.

After 3 months one would think that Connie had acquired an appetite inducing medication he could prescribe because of her pregnancy. Connie tried to force herself to eat and yet she had no appetite. At this point Connie's family was very worried about her and the unborn baby. Steve had spoken to his older sister about Connie's problem and his sister suggested that he give her a little marijuana to smoke to induce hunger and see if it works for Connie's lack of appetite. It took a lot of convincing by Steve to get Connie to try smoking it. She tried it and didn't like it the first time but the second time she tried it, the marijuana had induced hunger in Connie and she ate all her dinner and went back for seconds. It had worked.

After a month Connie's Doctor has seen a dramatic increase in body weight and was happily surprised and took full credit for her weight turn around. Of cause he wasn't the reason. It was the marijuana that had induce Connie's appetite. When Connie was in the Doctor's office and he was called out of the office she saw the name at the top and next to it was the word Pregorexic. It took her a minute or two to understand what that word meant. She didn't know whether she should tell the Doctor that her increase in normal body weight was due to taking marijuana. She felt he might disapprove of her taking marijuana as an appetite inducer. So she decided not to inform him. Connie went the full turn and gave birth to a 8lb. baby boy perfect. Connie and Steve would soon be married and raise their son together.

Lilly C. suffers from ANOREXIA NERVOSA

Lilly C. is a 32 year old Japanese female who has lived in the United States since age 15. She lives with her parents and younger brother. Lilly's father is a businessman who commutes between Japan and the United States, using a work visa for himself and his family. Lilly works part time in a bank and attends a Japanese school three afternoons each week to maintain her Japanese language skills. Lilly and her brother are fluently bilingual, her parents have some difficulty speaking in English. Lilly has been diagnosed with anorexia nervosa, a disorder that affects females with a drive towards thinness. Lilly is severely emaciated due to self- starvation and excessive exercise. She also has amenorrhea [stopping of menstrual periods]. Intense fear of gaining weight, extreme fatigue, social withdrawal and depression. She has received both a medical and a neurological evaluation to rule out a medical basis for her weight loss, and was determined to be suffering from anorexia nervosa.

Lilly experiences life threatening malnutrition, emaciation, low heart rate and blood pressure as well as hormonal and electrolyte impaired reasoning and severe fatigue. She is genuinely terrified of losing control over her eating and becoming overweight. Her perfectionism and desire to achieve correspond to a strong need for control also fears of inadequacy. Depression, and loss of esteem. Lilly is also experiencing cultural conflict in seeking to maintain her dual Japanese and American identities. Media and culture in both the United States and Japan glorify standards of thinness and beauty for females. Lilly was hospitalized on an eating disorder until in order to stabilize her medical condition and lay the foundation for outpatient treatment. During hospitalization Lilly was confined to bed during which time she was medically monitored, given fluids and electrolytes and given to option of tube feeding or eating on her own. She choose to eat on her own and made some progress with the gradual reintroduction of food. Once stabilized, Lilly was participating in group therapy where she learned she was not alone and was able to hear to experiences of others at varying stages of recovery. A behavioral contract guided her way toward some moderate weight gain. Her inpatient psychologist assisted Lilly in discharge planning by locating a Japanese American therapist with bilingual abilities. After Lilly's discharge she began individual therapy with family sessions as part of her treatment. She also decided to educate herself about her disease. She went to the library to get the information she needed and came across a book on herbs and herbal remedies.

She read about medical marijuana and other herbs and decided to try in a tea. It's been 4 years later after she tried the medical marijuana that her life has changed for the better. She was able to develop behavioral strategies with her psychologist to assist with decision making, thought stopping and reexamining her attitudes and expectations. When Lilly's depression and weight gain improved she was referred to a psychiatrist and put on low dose antidepressant medication. Her family was vital to her treatment, her concerns were discussed and she found her parents very respectful and attentive to her feelings. Her parents were encouraged to support her decisions and allow her to take steps toward independence while learning that her parents would neither condemn or abandon her. The family was able to discuss the challenges of dual American and Japanese identities' Lilly's family doesn't really agree with her use of medical marijuana, they support her use of it because they see how far she's come and all the great improvements in her treatment. Lilly's treatment went extremely smoothly in comparison to the many cases of anorexia nervosa. She bases this to the use of medical marijuana. Her individual therapy and medication treatment continued for three full years, as she gradually overcame her anorexia, she developed psychological, social and family resources.

Testimonials - Other Eating Disorders

Nanci G. suffers from MULTIPLE ILLNESSES

A beautiful 27 year old female model named Nanci G. is suffering from a combination of problems. Depression, anorexia nervosa, changes in her sleeping pattern, feeling worthless, sadness, loss of interest in activities, a fear of losing her status as a model to a younger model. Body weight loss due to not eating. Nanci's family gave her support and convinced her to seek help which she did. After seeing several doctors for depression and anorexia nervosa and therapy she fund that she did not like the affects of the medications that were prescribed. She remembered when she was a teenager and tried marijuana and it's affects like putting her in a positive attitude and making her feel hungry. Nanci began to buy marijuana an took small amounts and after several weeks she gained 10 pounds and is doing better with her modeling profession. She is still seeing the doctors and therapist every month. Nanci began to feel better about herself and less worried about her appearance and began to lose her depression slowly. Nanci began to examine herself and her own flows in herself so that she may correct them one by one. Nanci held off from entering in a relationship with any man until she felt confident enough to deal with another person. Nanci would go to a gym to exercise, bike riding, bowling and love to play video games. She soon met a man and began to date him. She realized he was not Mr. right but Mr. right now and not Mr. later. He would do for now and there would be others in the future in the quest for Mr. right. The quest goes on.

Elizabeth S. suffers from MULTIPLE ILLNESSES

Elizabeth S. suffers from Meningitis when she was a child. Elizabeth is 46 years old with a past history of ailments such as the Lupus disease, Bulimia nervosa, Anorexia nervosa.

Elizabeth has a combination of ailments which all can be treated and cured except Lupus. As far as Bulimia and Anorexia nervosa she has overcome these ailments with counseling and therapy. As for Lupus disease it would be a lifelong battle without end. The Lupus disease affects Elizabeth every day, it travels though her body affecting organs, joints and her immune system. One day her hands would swell up the next day it would be her knees and the day after that it would be a different joint in her body that was affected. She goes through monthly blood testing to track the disease. After one of these blood test it was discovered that her blood was thickening and she needed different medicine. Elizabeth had beaten the Bulimia nervosa problem but the Anorexia nervosa could flare up at any time triggered by a bout of depression. Elizabeth knows that in order for her to survive these ailments she must keep up her appetite and eat healthy foods. She would take marijuana for several reasons. It would increase her appetite to eat, relax her and help her deal with the pain, swelling and discomfort of the Lupus disease. It also picks up her mood when she felt mental depression coming on. Most of Elizabeth's time is spent dealing with the Lupus disease especially since it affects her immune system. To protect the immune system by eating nitrous foods, vitamins, herbs and minerals. Any disease that affects ones immune system can be potentially deadly and is very carious. The Lupus disease is not as well known as a disease such as AIDS or Cancer but it can be equally as deadly. There is no known cause for the Lupus disease or no known cure for it. Elizabeth must maintain her body weight and not fall back into Bulimia nervosa or Anorexia nervosa states. There for she must keep a positive attitude being that she is in a cause and effect situation regarding her ailments.

John I. suffers from an EATING DISORDER

John I. suffers from an eating disorder. His eating disorder is not anorexia nervosa but similar in one aspect. John does not eat enough food to put on body weight or maintain his normal weight. Some people are people that like to eat and enjoy eating food. They may have a normal appetite internal clock that lets them know when they are hungry and time to eat food. John is the opposite of this, he is not an eater. He does not enjoy eating foods, he does not have a normal appetite internal clock that functions properly. He eats just to sustain his life. He has to remind himself to eat something every day or he doesn't get hungry and has no appetite. John also has what's called a high energy metabolism burn. His body metabolism burns more energy than what he takes in. John is now 23 years old and living on his own. Before that, he lived with his parents in the house where he was raised as a child. Living at home his mother always saw to it that John ate at meal time because she knew that her son was not a good eater. When he was a child his mother always made him eat his food before he did anything else. Now that he is living by himself without his mother's coaching him to eat. He has to remember that he has to eat every day. John has been living on his own for only two years now and he realize now how difficult it is and stressful to live by one's self . With a low paying job, in a one bedroom apartment and not having the conveyance that he use to have at his parents' house. John has always been a slight young man and was considered a nerd amongst his parse. Not into much sports but keeps active. John spends his spear time by reading books, watching TV and playing video games. At times he would become stressed out over his problems. He would smoke marijuana as a appetite inducer and stress reliever. He would eat fat food all the time after he smoked marijuana May be some day John's internal hunger clock will be activated on its own but until then he would continue to take marijuana as a appetite inducer as well as some times other herbal medicines like onions, Angelica Archangelica, may apple, American mandrake.,.

Testimonials - Diabetes Mellitus

John W. suffers from DIABETES MELLITUS

John W. is a 61 year old that has diabetes mellitus (a disorder characterized by hyperglycemia and glyconsuria, resulting from inadequate production of insulin). He's a middle age man that's over weight does not exercise or eat the correct foods. Loves to drink beer and alcohol now must make a choice. Either to change his life style or possibly loose his life. So he choose to change his life style by exercising to lose weight. Eat low fat foods and no sugar products at all. Take medication and insulin as prescribed from his doctors. He began taking vitamins, minerals, proteins, and carbohydrates in his diet which will enable him to lose weight. Being a retired person having a lot of time on his hands he would take long walks and work in his house and garden. He began to cultivate marijuana along with other herbs, vegetables and flowers.

Immune Disorders

HIV and AIDS

PEOPLE SUFFERING WITH AIDS

A person having AIDS is always thinking about how much time they have to live. How long or short it may be. AIDS is a debilitating disease that attacks the immune system and in doing so lowering the bodies resistance to viruses. With this disease even a common cold could be life threatening. AIDS patients have been unfairly stigmatized by other ignorant people that are not a wear of the patient's problems. AIDS is still on the rise all over the world. There has been reported from Africa five million new infected people in the past year and three million died the year before. There are some new AIDS fighting medications on the market that are helping prolong life. In this country many AIDS patients will take medical marijuana to ease their discomfort and pain. Acquired Immune Deficiency Syndrome is on the rise worldwide. All races and ethnic groups are affected this disease does not discriminate. In the past 20 years many AIDS patients will take medical marijuana to increase appetite and as a discomfort relaxer. Even though AIDS patients should not smoke they have taken marijuana mixed in tea and salads. Some other herbal medicine for treating AIDS are Aloe Gel, Ashwagandha, Asian Ginseng, Chaparral, Chinese Cucumber, Codonopsis, Astragalus, Schisandra, Milk Vetch, Balsam Pear, and many others. Crohn's Disease etiology is unknown, and research examining the role of immune factors, infectious agents, and dietary factors. After having a subcutaneous mastectomy for the chronic disease called Fibrocystic Breast disease, the patient will go through many adjustments to the new situation. Many women that have had this surgery will take medical marijuana as a pick me up medication. Agitated depression is a psychiatric depression that symptoms are restlessness, feelings of guilt, depressed, phobias, crying, agitated obsessions and ideas of being persecuted. This is very similar to manic depressive patients. Meningitis virus causes loss of appetite which is treated with medical marijuana put in tea so that the patient does not get a headache. To beat this virus the patient must eat food in order to maintain strength.

AIDS and other illnesses

Kaposi's Sarcoma associated opportunistic infections and the immune suppression associated with AIDS. Leukemia in adults has four different forms. Marijuana is taken as a appetite inducer for weight loss and anorexia. Herpes Zoster otherwise known as Shingles which is theorized that varicella zoster virus lies dormant in the dorsal root ganglia and is reactivated by and acute illness or emotional stress, trauma, systemic disease like Hodgkin disease. Some people over 50 years old and people who are HIV positive are more likely to develop the disease. Marijuana is taken as a relaxer medication.

Sickle Cell Anemia is an ongoing illness that's debilitating physically as well as mentally. It has been reported that adults afflicted with this illness are taking medical marijuana mixed in teas and mixed in to salads for ingestion Ankylosing Spondylitis affects more men than women, affecting the spinal column and joints. People that are affected with this disease feel pain in there lower back area as well as limited motion in affected joints and lumbar spine. The patient will experience stiffness in the morning, back pain, weight loss. None steroidal anti inflammatory drugs to reduce pain, spasm, and swelling and to facilitate exercise are usually prescribed. It has been reported that a large number of these patient are taking medical marijuana to increase their appetite and deal with the pain. Scoliosis curvature of the spine can give chronic pain on a daily bases. Some people live with some form of scoliosis that does not affect daily lives. There are a few forms of glaucoma disease which affects the optic nerve. Chronic glaucoma patients might have enlargement of anterior culinary veins, dilated pupils, pain, poor vision during an attack. The visual field may be normal. Marijuana cannot cure this disease but it can help the patient cope with the disease. Reiter's syndrome affects men only. It appears as a nonspecific urethritis. The symptoms include arthritis and conjunctivitis. A large spectrum of antibiotics are used for treating urethritis. Pain therapy an medications are used and some patients will take medical marijuana as one of the medications. Collagen diseases affect the bodies connective tissue or soft skeleton. The supporting tissue of various organs, blood vessels, joints contain lesions.

Those people that have AIDS have but one thought on their minds is to survive this somewhat new disease. Outside of changing ones physical being it changes ones mental condition as well. A person having AIDS is always thinking about how much time they have to live. How long or short it may be. AIDS is a debilitating disease that attacks the immune system and in doing so lowering the bodies resistance to viruses. With this disease even a common cold could be life threatening. AIDS patients have been unfairly stigmatized by other ignorant people that are not aware of the patient's problems. AIDS is still on the rise all over the world. There has been reported from Africa five million new infected people in the past year and three million died the year before. There are some new AIDS fighting medications on the market that are helping prolong life. In this country many AIDS patients will take marijuana to ease their discomfort and pain. Acquired Immune Deficiency Syndrome is on the rise worldwide. All races and ethnic groups are a affected this disease does not discriminate. In the past 20 years many AIDS patients have take marijuana mixed in tea and in salads. Some other herbal medicine for treating AIDS are, Aloe Gel, Ashwagandha, Asian Ginseng, Chaparral, Chinese Cucumber, Codonopsis, Astragals, Schisandra, Milk Vetch, Balsam Pear, and many others.

Alan H. has AIDS

Alan H. is suffering with acquired immunodeficiency syndrome (AIDS), for the past 3 years. At this point it makes no difference how Alan got the human immunodeficiency virus (HIV) that causes AIDS. What does matter is how Alan deals with the illness to stay alive. Alan has been undergoing treatment for AIDS that is enhancing his survival and quality of life. AIDS has become a major worldwide epidemic, the most advanced stages of HIV infection. There are more than 7000,000 cases of AIDS have been reported in the United States and as many as 900,000 Americans may be infected with HIV. The epidemic is growing most rapidly among the minority populations and women. Alan is so debilitated by the symptoms AIDS that he cannot hold steady employment or do house hold chores. He experience phases of intense life threatening illness followed by phases in which he functions normally. Alan is currently taking antiretroviral drugs to fight HIV infection and its associated infections. Alan takes medical marijuana mainly as a appetite inducer to help him keep his body weight up. One of the effects from AIDS is weight loss and lack of the appetite Alan also said that medical marijuana helps relax him when he has bouts of depression or stress. Alan's gets help from his family and friends to serve his needs. Medical marijuana can be taken in conjunction with other antiretroviral without conflict or hang over. Alan has his good days and has his bad days and always is optimistic about living and yet he gave the impression that if he didn't live that was all right to. He understood that we all are born to die, and it's just a matter of when.

Dan G has HIV

Dan G. has Human Immunodeficiency Virus (HIV) positive for four years at the age of 35. Some of Dan's symptoms related to the AIDS is weight loss, sleepless nights, depression, and AIDS Dementia. Last year Dan was treated for pneumonia that was treated successfully. Dan seemed a little withdrawn. A long with Dan's medications he would take medical marijuana to help him deal with the AIDS. Dan is a X- drug addict, that become HIV positive with an infected needle. He was able to beat his drug addiction and now he is battling AIDS. Dan knows that marijuana is illegal in his State but at the point in his life the legalities do not matter. All that matters to Dan is survival. To survive this disease the best way Dan can. Dan is not working due to the illness and is being provided for by the State assistance programs. Dan would spend a lot of time playing his guitar and writing and creating music. He thinks that he doesn't have much time so he pushes himself to write more music. There are many times he doesn't have the energy to even pick up his guitar or even get out of bed. Dan smokes medical marijuana and hour before eating food. In doing this it helps his appetite. Dan had very few friends before he was infected with the virus. And after getting the virus he has none. Even thaw times are changing some things remain the same. Like some peoples attitude regarding AIDS.

Dan realized that not many people want to be friend a person with AIDS. He didn't like being along after all; he always had someone to hang out with, but not now. So he decided to place a ad in the news paper dating section, stating that he was HIV positive and he is seeking a HIV positive female. Dan was feeling lonely and needing companionship. It took him some time to place the ad but he did. He has a answering machine hooked up to his phone so he could monitor incoming calls and record and play back the calls. It didn't take long before Dan had gotten responses from his ad. He had gotten three responses from three different women that were HIV positive themselves. Dan listened to all three responses over and over again to analyze the most compatible. Dan chose two out of the three women to talk to over the phone for a few days before meeting them in person. Dan had arranged face to face dates with both women on different days. This went on for several weeks of talking to both women and dating both women. Dan couldn't afford to continue to take out the two women so he had to make a decision on which women would be number one. One of the women made the decision for him by telling him that she just wanted to be friends and nothing else. The woman that Dan stayed with was a good choice. They had a lot in common and got along well together as well as helped each other deal with their illnesses. They both checked on each other to make sure each other was taking their medications and keeping doctor appointments. They would both smoke medical marijuana before meal time as an appetite inducer. There is the old saying; there is someone for everyone in the world.

David B. suffers from AIDS

David B. suffers from AIDS at the age of 32 years old and has been dealing with it for the past four years with treatment and medications to fight the virus. Although David has physical problems he also has severe stress that effects him physiologically and impairs his body's ability to fight off invading viruses and bacteria. This stress just adds to the weakening of his body's immune system in conjunction with the AIDS virus. The psychosocial stress factor is having a effect on the functional status in his immune system and makes it difficult to treat the HIV.

Psychosocial stressors and his mental state has depress immune function to the point as to make him more vulnerable to viruses, bacteria and germs. Episodes of depression that are triggered by stress and a difficult life events or side effects of medications, or the effects of HIV on his brain. Depression limits the energy needed to keep focused on staying healthy. David is not working at this time and pays his bills with money he receives from the Government and disability payments. David has a few friends that he can count on and many that he can't. Many of his family and friends have disassociated themselves from him. Never the less he has learned who his real friends are and who he could trust. David always says it's not his time to go yet and he will continue to fight for his life until he can't fight any more. The illness at times leaves David weak as a kitten and he gets stressed out over it and not being able to do any of his daily activities. Soon after he would fall in to a state of depression. David would take marijuana in tea or smoke it in a pipe. It had a up lifting effect and seemed to relax his stress and increase his appetite which helped him to eat more food to build his body and immune system.

David spends a lot of time at Doctors offices, clinics, hospitals, and places that provide the treatment for HIV. A psychotherapist prescribes talk therapy to help as well.

Prescription antidepressant medications were also added. David would live from day to day not looking to the future and yet he still has hope. There are many people with AIDS that don't have any family or other people that they can count on for help in times of need. That's why there are so many places that a lone person can get help when needed, if the person knows where to get the help. In almost every State there is some place where a person with AIDS can get help, whether it be physical help or mental help. There are clinics, consolers, talk groups, hospitals that have care and therapy to treat the problem. There are even on line web sites that give a tremendous amount of information to help a person with AIDS. Some people like David need someone to guide him to the best alternative to help him. David is very hopeful about all the new medicines on the market and believes some day there will be a cure for AIDS but until then he will try anything that prolongs his life.

Megan suffers from AIDS

Megan is a 27 year old single women that's an accountant in a large stock exchange company. She recently was diagnosed with AIDS, she was in shock for a long time. After going through the gilt stage and why me stage she began to focus on her health and how and when she acquired HIV. Megan investigated and contacted all her current and previous sexual partners within a selective time period. This was very hard and embarrassing to do but it had to be done. This disease had changed her life in every way. These day's the medical world has made great strides in AIDS medicines to prolong life for HIV patients. As long as she continued to take the AIDS medication and kept a good diet she would survive it. She began to practice abstinence pertaining to sex for fear of spreading the disease. She went to counseling and a support group for help. Megan soon realized she had only one or two real friends that she could count on. After acquiring HIV she soon found out who her real friends were and who was not. One of the real friends that she had was Pat who went to school with. Megan and Pat had been very close. Pat had moved out of the area for several years and retuned and help her friend that was ill. Pat would on occasion take on what's called the girl's night out to a night club to go dancing and have a good time. Pat notice that Megan was not eating properly or enough food due to a lack of appetite. Pat suggested to Megan that she needs an appetite inducer to increase Megan's appetite. Megan had remember when she was a teenager and had tried marijuana and how hungry it had made her. She had purchased some marijuana. Almost at once she began to eat more, and gain body weight and her attitude became more positive and hopeful. She also took herbal medicines for AIDS like Aloe Gel, Astragalus to improve immunity and several others.

Sarah R. suffers from HIV

Sarah R. is 37 years old married with two teenage children that lives in a suburban middle class neighborhood. Her husband's name is Ron who is a department store manager at one of the bigger shopping Malls. Sarah works part time as a telephone operator and the other time she was a devoted mother and wife and home maker. She was happy and content with her life and family until one day. Sarah's job at the telephone company required a mandatory physical check up every 5 years so Sarah went for a checkup thinking she to herself that it was time to get a check up any way. When she received the results of the test the doctor requested that she take some more test which made Sarah wonder why. After the second set of test came back from the lab the doctor called Sarah to come into his office to talk about the results. When Sarah arrived at the doctor's office he had informed her that she was HIV positive and she went into immediate shock. The doctor requested that she take more test and refer her to other specialist.

Whenever Sarah had a major problem she would go to this particular public park in her area in which she spent most of her youth at. In the park there was a small lake and a small Gazebo near it in which she would go sit in for hours on end. She would think over the problem in this atmosphere of calm and peace and come to a solution of the problem. As in the past Sarah went to the Gazebo for hours racking her brains on how she could have gotten HIV. She knows that she was not have sex with anyone except her husband Ron. She at first refused to believe that her husband Ron had anything to do with it so she began to think if she could have gotten HIV elsewhere like her job or in basic contact with something like and open cut or hand rail or toilet bowl seat. None of these things was the cause of how she got it, she had concluded. She is slowly realizing that her whole life would change because of this.

Sarah decided not to inform her husband and children of her illness until she had gotten more information about how and when she had gotten HIV and how to treat it. Sarah from then on had changed but she would act like everything was normal and still the same as always. Sarah is a good actress when she has to. Sarah's doctor recommended that she inform her family to get there support but Sarah was not ready yet to tell them until she had more answers. Her doctor had said that she should contact any and all persons that she had sexual contact with. In her mind that only meant her husband Ron so she hired a private investigator to get information on her husband's actions. Within one week the investigator had proof of many different affairs that her husband Ron had with other women. Sarah had confronted Ron about what she had found out about his different affairs as well as her contracting AIDS from him as a carrier of this disease. Sarah demanded that Ron leave the house until she decided what to do next. She knew what was next and that was to tell her children about this new changing situation.

After a few months the disease and depression began to affect Sarah, feeling sick and betrayed by her husband Ron. She began to go for treatment for the illness and treatment for depression as well, at an HIV clinic and AIDS counseling. The children have adapted well to the situation and are excepting the changes in all their lives. The children still had a deep routed anger for their fathers betrayal and the consequence of his selfish actions. Sarah started to concentrate on fighting this disease and keeping a positive attitude about her situation and try to stay strong. She began to take some new AIDS fighting medications as well as vitamins and minerals, healthy foods, herbal medicines. Sarah received a large divorce settlement for her and child support for the children and yet she still was depressed and unhappy. She started to try to get her life back together again after feeling it had been destroyed. Sarah began to go out on dates but nothing steady with any one man. She was afraid of passing HIV on to someone else. At one of the AIDS counseling sessions Sarah met a man named Mark that was HIV positive to. He acquired HIV due to a bad blood needle transfusion. He was attracted to Sarah and would ask her out on dates. Sarah and Mark would take marijuana to increase their appetites along with other medicines and medications. Sarah slowly started to get her life back together again. The marijuana also helped Sarah with her depression.

Richard C. suffers from AIDS

Richard C. suffers from having AIDS for the past three years. Undergoing radiation treatment ad drugs to battle the virus. These days most of us know what AIDS is and know of the symptoms and effects. Richard was prescribed medical marijuana by one of his doctors with a prescription but due to all the red tape in filling the prescription Richard started to buy marijuana from dealers and friends. He would use it to ease his stress and pick up his appetite for food to build back up his body. It helps him deal with this life threatening disease. Richard became a medical marijuana cultivator by learning how to grow it in his spare time. For Richard the thought of not knowing how much time he has to live out ways the risk of being arrested for drug possession for growing it. Richard learned how to grow the plants so that they did not look like marijuana. He had cultivated it to look like Japanese bonsai plants. After a short period of time it became a hobby or common alliance between where Richard would water and feed his plants and the plants would return medication. Richard would still go through AIDS test and test medicines. He's going for radiation treatment and steroids treatment for weight loss. Richard was no longer sexually active for fear of spreading the AIDS virus. Richard would have his good feeling and have his bad feeling days. Hopefully the new AIDS fighting drugs make a difference in helping Richard fight the AIDS disease. No one knows how much time each one of us has to live that's why we should live each day like it is our last day alive. Richard would eat more natural and notorious foods, vitamins, and minerals. The AIDS disease as far as Richard's concerned it has stabilized for now. He also would take other herbal medicines like Asian Ginseng, Astragalus, Balsam, Pear, Schisandra.

Testimonials - Lyme Disease and Tuberculosis

Margret T suffers from LYME DISEASE

Margret T. is a 40 year old mother of two that is suffering from Lyme Disease. Margret's two children are in there twenties and in college. Margret's husband works part time and when not at work he's home helping out. It is believed that Margret had acquired the Lyme Disease three years prior on a vacation trip at a country resort. Somewhere during that vacation Margret was infected with spirochete, probably transmitted by deer ticks. At first Margret thought she had the flu or a virus and went to her doctor for an examination. When her blood test and other test came back from the lab, she was diagnosed with advanced Lyme Disease and was hospitalized. When the disease was in remission Margret was sent home and was monitored as a outpatient. She would continue to see her neurologist to see how much the Lyme Disease had affected her nervous system. After a year Margret was diagnosed with Osteo Neurogenic Arthritis following after the Lyme Disease. Margret would take numerous medications to relieve the joint pain and inflammation,. Some worked and some did not. She also would take herbal medication like medical marijuana, German chamomile, ginger, ginseng, elderberry, and Kava for stress and tension. In the interview Margret would not say where she got the medical marijuana and I didn't ask.

James H. suffering from TURBERCULOSIS

James H. suffering from Tuberculosis (TB) for 10 years dealing with the disease on a daily basis. He is a 62 year old retired plumber living off S.S.I. and a small retirement pension. James lives by himself with no family or relatives to help him. He has a home attendant 3 to 4 times a week and a house keeper 3 times a week. James long time friend Willy would visit James watching sports events on cable TV and talking about current news events, play video games, chess, cards and pool. James would also have Willy bring marijuana to help him with his ailments. James and Willy would never share anything that might possibly spread Tuberculosis to Willy so James was always extra careful. Everything in James's home is constantly being sterilized. James takes many medications for the disease, some help him and some don't. Marijuana helps him medically and yet in his State it is illegal. Illegal or not, James says that marijuana helps him make it through the day. One day at a time. James H. pasted away in 2004.

<u>Musculoskeletal Disorders</u>

JOINT DISORDERS

Inflammation of the joints accompanied by pain and swelling which is the M.O. of arthritis, arthritis can come from a number of conditions including infection like tuberculosis, rheumatic fever, trauma, ulcerative colitis, degenerative joint disease as osteoarthritis, metabolic disturbances as gout. Rheumatoid arthritis is a systemic disease of unknown cause characterized by inflammatory changes in joints, swelling and can be chronic. Degenerative arthritis is a progressive joint disease involving multiple joints, characterized by destruction of joint cartilage and other degenerative changes, usually affecting the elderly. If one never had any form of arthritis it may be hard for them to understand the amount of pain and discomfort on a constant basis. Having certain forms of arthritis can be debilitating and crippling that effects the person's emotions, thinking, total health and life style. Some people that have arthritis have it in the milder forms and do not have arthritic attacks as frequently as the more aggressive types of arthritis. These people will say things like it must be going to rain today because my leg or arm or shoulder is paining me today. In some cases the change in climate and weather conditions may be the cause of their flair up. For more aggressive types of arthritis the patient will us medical marijuana in conjunction with a bee sting on the inflamed area. There is an organic substances in the stinger of the bee that when injected into the affected area over rides the pain in that area. Arthritis affects more than 50 million Americans, men and women are equally affected. The other types of herbal medicines that are recommended to treat these ailments are American Ginseng, Chondroitin, Elderberry, Kava, Burdock, Guggui, SAMe, Slippery Elm, and many more. Nearly 50 million Americans have some form of arthritis although there is no cure affective treatments are available. Osteoarthritis affects nearly 21 million Americans, and old injury to one or more joints at an early age also may lead to osteoarthritis years later. Excessive stressful use of joints over years may cause osteoarthritis in those joints later on. Some old injuries might heal inadequately resulting in a lump. This develops in people over the age of 45 years old. Almost all Americans older than 60 years old have mild symptoms of osteoarthritis in a joint before or during a change in the weather is one of the signs as well swelling and stiffness in a joint.

Arthritis, Osteoarthritis, and Other Disorders

Most bursitis is unknown, although trauma, arthritis, gout, and infection have been implicated. Tenderness around a shoulder accompanied by limited range of motion as well as swelling and pain. The Gout mainly affects middle age and older men. This disease shows signs of acute arthritis and inflammation of the joints. It will usually start in the feet and knees and begins to increase pain gradually at night time. Thousands of men are affected with this disease on a daily bases. People will take different medications an treatments for pain relief. Medical marijuana is taken as one of the pain treatments used by many. Many people that were athletic in their younger lives are now affected with gout as well as people with old injures. Gout has been around for ages and has had many different treatments from hot compresses to pain killers to sleeping pills as well as marijuana as for pain relief an sleeping aid. Stiff men syndrome and stiff women syndrome are affected with intermittent tightness, aching, and stiffness of muscles.

Some patients are taking marijuana as a relaxer. The gout is recurrent, acute arthritis of the peripheral joints, particularly the great toe. Repeated acute attacks lead to chronic arthritis. Tendinitis and Tenosynovitis are characterized by pain when the joints is moving, repetitive movement, strain, or excessive exercise may be the cause. Systemic diseases may also be the cause like rheumatoid arthritis, gout, sclerosis, infections. Adults over the age of 40 years old and athletes or people with jobs requiring repetitive movement are more likely to acquire tendinitis. It has been reported that some people with tendinitis are taking marijuana to treat the pain and discomfort as well as a relaxer. Temporomandibular Joint Syndrome disorder include congenital and development anomalies like joint disease like arthritis, ankylosis, neoplasm's, or Lupus. The jaw could have been dislocated from a trauma or fracture, teeth clenching or grinding and prolonged stress. Fractures and dislocations produce a shift in the mandible which leads to asymmetric jaw movements, muscle spasms, and pain. Limited jaw movement causes pain. Marijuana is taken to relieve pain and stress and to induce relaxation.

Nearly 40 million Americans have some form of arthritis although there is no cure affective treatment are available. Osteoarthritis affects nearly 21 million Americans . An old injury to one or more joints at an early age also may lead to osteoarthritis in those joints later on. Some old injuries might heal inadequately resulting in a lump. This develops in people over the age of 45 years old. Almost all Americans older than 60 years old have mild symptoms of osteoarthritis in a joint before or during a change in the weather is one of the signs as well as swelling and stiffness in a joint.

People with herniated disk have great back pain the lumber hernia ion is most common and generally occurs in adults 20 to 45 years of age. Men are affected more often than women. The main feature is pain in the lower back going down one leg or pain in the neck that goes down one arm. Some patients after having back surgery will take marijuana relaxant and to relieve a person's base line pressure. Its estimated that 69 to 85 million Americans have hypertension. Marijuana is taken as a relaxer.

Testimonials - Bursitis

Abraham D. suffers from BURSITIS

Abraham D. is a 45 year old manager that suffers from Bursitis in his shoulder and some times in his knees. The cause of this Bursitis was from doing 20 years of manual labor at constriction work sites. Abraham gets cortisone injections whenever the Bursitis is overwhelming to him. He also was affected with Osteoarthritis which affected his hands and other discriminating joint areas of his body. This joint disease impaired the movement function due to inflammation of the joint cartilage. Abraham is also receiving treatment for this debilitating disease and medications. His family is very supportive of him and his illness. Having a managerial job enabled him to still work without doing physical labor. Although here are times when the illnesses affect his legs and he is unable to walk without having pain. Some days Abraham will use a walking cane, usually more days than less days. He spends a large amount of time at his doctors office, the arthritis clinic, physical therapy and pain therapy. Abraham would complain to his doctor of lack of sleep due to pain discomfort so the doctor prescribed a night time pain pill medication which would work but it left Abraham groggy and lethargic in the morning and would take several hours to dissipate. So he went back to his doctor who prescribed a lesser dosage pain pill medication.

The Bursitis would flair up more when there were changes in the weather. When there was an approaching rain storm the climate would change and affect his joints which led to pain and discomfort. Abraham would take marijuana for additive pain relieve in conjunction with his other pain medications which was comparable to each other and not conflicting. Abraham could only work as a manager part time in the family business. His family was wealthy and would help him financially when he needed it. When Abraham was much younger he would look down on all the young people of his time that were taking marijuana for non medicinal use. He said then that he would never take marijuana. One thing he has learned is, never say never. No one can product the future even though they think they can. He at one time stated that marijuana had alleviated the vexation feelings that he had and relaxed him. He also would take other herbal medicines like Ashwagandha, Chondritin, Devil's Claw, Glucosamine, Slippery Elm and Asian Ginseng, As time moves on Abraham began to feel better but not cured.

Kurt S. suffers from BURSITIS

Kurt S. is a 45 year old construction manager that suffers from Bursitis in his shoulder due from working many years in construction. He also is and x-alcoholic for 10 years. Kurt has been taking medical marijuana for several years to help with his Bursitis and alcoholism. Kurt has tried every kind of shoulder pain medication on the market and under the sun and still will state that marijuana eases his shoulder pain along with other mild pain medications best. Kurt has said that in the state in which he lives in there is no programs available for medical marijuana to treat different medical illnesses. He does not like to feel like he has to break the law to purchase marijuana to treat his illness but he feels he has to do what's best for himself. Kurt found out that in the past like in the 1970's there were such state programs pertaining to medical marijuana used to treat medical illnesses. Such programs state wide were allowed to end and not be reinstated in the 1980's due to the very powerful drug companies lobbing against it. He hopes someday soon that the state and Federal Gov, will have legalization of medical marijuana for the treatment of illnesses. There are thousands of people with medical illnesses that want the same in their states and some day the Gov. and states will have programs that allow people with medical illnesses to take medical marijuana legally.

ARTHRITIS MUSCULAR RHEUMATISM

Muscular Rheumatism Fibrositis is inflammation of white fibrous connective tissue anywhere in the body. Symptoms are soreness and stiffness of muscles, and pain in joints and spasm. Includes such conditions as Fibromyositis,. Myositis, Myalgia,. People that have had attacks of Rheumatic Fever which is systemic, febrile disease that's inflammatory variable in severity and duration. Later gives rise to periodical discomfort and joint pain when in motion. Soft tissue rheumatism is pain around joints but which are not related to or caused by joint disease. The everyday terms for these are Bursitis, Tennis Elbow, Tendinitis, Stiffman Syndrome. Many veteran sports athletes suffer from these ailments. Rheumatoid arthritis can strike at any time but usually develops between the ages 20 and

50 years old. It is estimated that 2 million people have rheumatoid arthritis, twice as many women as men are affected. Pain and swelling in the smaller joints of your hands and feet, aching or Stiffness of the joints and muscles. Loss of motion and strength in muscles attached to the affected joints. Many patients will take marijuana to treat their pain and discomfort.

Other herbal medicines are also taken like Asian Ginseng, Ashwagandha, Elderberry, Glucosamine, Kava, Pychgenol, and others. Everyone has had anxious moments in their life whether good moments or bad moments. It is normal to have anxiety neurosis. Anxiety neurosis is a functional disease which symptoms are somatic thoughts of fear that are manifested out of proportion to extreme fear and frustration out of proportion can lead to anxiety state. A person with this disease can experience asymptomatic complains like heart pain, head aces, nerves cold, hot, sweaty an other symptoms. This is not a physical disease or organic disease but a mental disorder which is treatable. Another form of this disorder is anxious agitated depression which symptoms are lack of sleep, depression, agitation, worry, delusions, panic. There have been reports indicating that people are taking medical marijuana to treat these illnesses. As well as other herbal medicines like American Ginseng, Asian Ginseng, Ashwagandha, Gotu KAVA, St. John Wort, and many others. Marijuana can also be used for weight loss with the proper diet, and exercise. Naturally the overweight person would have to change their eating habits and food intake. Marijuana sometimes has the opposite effect of increasing appetite with certain individuals. Lenex W. is 29 years old and overweight. He had made up his mind to loss the excess weight by dieting and excise on a daily bases. His routine was a small breakfast go to work and at lunch time fruits and salad. After work go to the gym. For an hour or two and then go home for dinner which was small portions of food. He would take medical marijuana as a relax activator. With his system he lost the amount of weight he wanted to.

Carcinoma, scirrhus, epithelioma, are just other names for Cancer. We all know about cancer and what a devastating disease and what it does to the body and mind. When a person first finds out they have cancer their whole life changes as well as their mental state. As time moves on about ten months of going through the barrage of cancer treatments and tests drugs and radiation treatment. The person will start to look for alternative treatment and medications to combat the illness. Some might be vitamins, medicines, organic herbal products. One of the basic first treatment in a hospital is to make the patient comfortable as possible and to serve four to six small meals and try to stimulate the appetite the patient. They try to keep the patient cheerful and upbeat. As a part of the disease is loss of weight and appetite amongst other associated problems.

One of the main side effects is loss of appetite due to cancer fighting test drugs. Marijuana has been taken by cancer patients as a appetite inducer. It Is accentual that the cancer patient's body receives good amounts of nutritional foods to build up there resistance against this debilitating disease. Other herbal medicines that are used: Aloe gei, Ashwagandha, Asian Ginseng, Astragalus, Chaparral, Mayapple, Pycnogenol, Reishi, Scullcap, Soy, and others.

Testimonials - Arthritis

Macy A. suffers from RHEUMATOID ARTHRITIS

Macy A. is suffering from Rheumatoid Arthritis. When she was younger she was a athlete that ran the 100 yard dash and several other sports events. The rheumatoid arthritis affects her knees and ankles and sometimes other parts of her body. Some of her symptoms are pain and swelling of her feet and knees, aching or stiffness of her joints and muscles. She had loss of motion in her legs due to the affected joints. Some time it affects all parts of her body. Her doctor had her take several blood test, rheumatoid factor test, C-reactive protein test, and Erythrocyte sedimentation rate test.. She was prescribed medications, and light exercises like Taichi for chronic pain. She would take medical marijuana as a relaxer for discomfort. Macy works in a Law office and is constantly at her work station for hours on end. She is a dedicated good worker and will do work over time to complete the task. Having to sit for hours in the same chair can be very painful or discomforting . Macy made her work station as comfortable as possible to not aggravate her knees. She has a special chair on wheels so to limit her movement like walking that may be painful on any given day.

When Macy gets home from work and after she has dinner, she will take her medication for the disorder and take medical marijuana as a relaxer and listen to music of a relaxing nature. Some days Macy has her good days and some are bad days. On her bad days a short trip to the local store can become a painful gauntlet of obstacles, like walking up a flight of stairs or driving a car in heavy traffic inducing stress and knee pain. Macy mostly uses public transportation and cabs. Macy would take medical marijuana sometimes every day if she had pain on those days. She said it helps her cope with her pain. She said she wishes she could have medical marijuana legally. Macy said she believes in the near future medical marijuana would be legal in all the United States. AFTER ALL THE TIMES ARE CHANGING EVEN NOW.

Macy's boy friend Dan has been seeing Macy for some time and he understands that medical marijuana helps Macy with her illness, and condones it even though he is a policeman. Dan being a policeman should be enforcing the law on marijuana with Macy but he won't. Dan believes that the laws pertaining to marijuana for medical use for patients with medical illnesses should be amended. He knows that Macy is taking marijuana for her pain that he sees she is in. Some other herbs used to treat Rheumatism and Arthritis: Devil's Claw, Harpagophytum, Salix, and Urtica, Boswellia sacra, Amica Montana, Chrysanthemum Parenium, Filipendula ulmaria.

Angela S has REITER'S SYNDROME

Angela S. is a 35 year old part time office worker that suffers b from a recurring virus called Reiter's syndrome (urethritritis, arthritis, and conjunctivitis). Angela takes many antibiotics when this virus reoccurs. She takes pain medication, medical marijuana, green tea, gingko, carrots, cod-liver oil, clove and a normal diet of foods. Angela said that she does not know how or where she the virus but she's dealing with it as a part of her life and refuses to give in to it. Angela being a quiet private young lady said that she wished that her

State had the legalization for medical marijuana in her State. She said that she hated the fact that every time she buys marijuana for medical use, that she is breaking the law. Angela said that some day when her State comes into the new century that marijuana will be allowed for medical use. But until then she will continue to buy marijuana illegally to treat her ailment.

Jason M. suffers from RHEUMATOID ARTHRITIS

Jason M. is 52 years old and is suffering from rheumatoid arthritis after having rheumatic fever when he was a child. He has dealt with mild forms of arthritis most of his life but this disease has affected different parts of his body. The joints in his hand would swell up and give him pain with discomfort as well as his knees. He would loss motion and their use. Jason's profession was a phone repairman but the advent of this disease left him no option but to go on disability. Being on disability meant he had less money to pay bills and he had to change his life style to adapt. Jason was divorced from his wife and his children are grown up. He lives alone in a one bedroom apartment. He now would have to budget his money to make ends meet. Part of the rheumatoid medications was paid for by insurance and the other part he had to pay for. He got a part time job as a security guard monitoring a security monitor in the evenings. As time moved on he began to get less sleep and eat less food and fall into a depression state of mind. His personality began to change due to the disease and lower life style. He had went to this rheumatologist who refer him to another doctor for treatment for depression. Sue was Jason's girl friend and helped when their schedules permitted for them to see each other. She would visit him a few days out of the week. She would cook for him and clean things in the place to help Jason specially when the arthritis was at its worst. Sue notice the change in Jason's mood, he began to have low self esteem or attitude and some signs of decreased mental and physical energy. Sue also noticed a decrease in his sexual drive and a loss of appetite as well as weight loss. Sue was not going to get there disease's destroy her relationship with Jason so she started to make plans on what to do to combat this.

She began to tackle it one step at a time, first finding information about the types of rheumatoid arthritis medication Jason was taking and finding out if they were the best choice's of drugs for Jason's needs. Whatever medication that was prescribe that proved in affective were discontinued and new medication was prescribed by the rheumatologist that helped. When a person has multiple disease's sometimes the drugs and medication's can conflict with each other or have an adverse reaction in the patient. The medication prescribed for depression was conflicting with the previous medication prescribed for rheumatologic arthritis All though Jason's arthritis pain was more manageable he still had loss of appetite and weight loss. She began to tackle this by cooking all of Jason's favorite foods and dishes but this had little effect on Jason's appetite. Sue decided to contact her younger sister Linda who was in the health field for information about the problem. Linda suggested that Jason look into some herbal products for better nutrition and health. Sue began to investigate about organically grown foods. Herbs and minerals for the both of them. Sue found out which herbal products are suited for their needs and perched them. After some time past they both felt better but Jason still loss of appetite and depression. Sue was about to give up when her sister Linda suggested to have Jason try marijuana to help his lack of appetite. In Jason and Sue's state there was no legal medical marijuana available for patients so they purchased marijuana through a friend. There are only 10 States in America that have legal programs for medical marijuana available for patients. Jason tried the marijuana and began to be more active physically as well as mentally. He began to eat more food and gain body weight. Sue also notice and increase in Jason's sexual drive. Jason began to improve more and more each day. The marijuana aided in conjunction with other medications to help Jason's illnesses. Some of the herbal medicines Jason is taking for (Ashwagandha) which is an Indian herbal equivalent to Ginseng, Elderberry, and Kava for stress and tension. He also took colchicum. Jason had herd on the news that some of the arthritis medicine increased the risk of heart attack or stroke by 50%. Jason was happy that he had discontinued there use and is taking more natural medicines and medications.

143

Fred S. suffers from Arthritis and Lupus

Fred S. Is a 65 year old factory manager with arthritis and lupus disease which is a bad combination. Lupus by itself has its own form of arthritis that has doubled with rheumatoid arthritis. Fred lost the use of his hands and control of his fingers. The lupus disease attacks different parts of his body at will on a daily bases. One day it will affect his feet or legs or arms. The next day it will affect a different part of his body like neck, or hands or other parts of his body. Fred's wife Millie had gotten a part time job to help out with their financial needs a little. Fred is mainly home or at one of three doctors offices for treatment or to fill prescriptions at the pharmacy. The lupus disease and rheumatoid arthritis had changed almost all the aspects of his life. The pain and discomfort at times was unbearable during the day time and at night time he had to take sleeping pills to sleep straight through the night. Lupus affects women 20 times more than men. Yet lupus is more rare in men than in women but it does occur. Lupus also affects the body's immune system in a similar fashion to the AIDS disease. Rheumatoid arthritis has similar symptoms to the lupus disease just more intense. There is no cure for the lupus disease or rheumatoid arthritis. One day in the future there will be a cure for lupus and many other life threatening diseases but until then there still must be tests for new cures and treatments for the elimination of these diseases. Fred would take marijuana with other herbal medicines for pain and discomfort and relaxation. Fred's wife Millie would make sure that Fred took his medication and had a good diet. Some rashes that occur on different parts of his body at different times. He also experiences headaches, depression, weakness, dizziness. Lupus is an autoimmune disease that is also known as a rheumatic disease that cause aches, pain, and stiffness in the joints, muscles, and bones. Fred has blood and urine tests every month to prevent kidney damage due to e lupus disease. Monitoring the central nervous system can be needed. These laboratory tests are used to monitor the progress of the disease once it has been diagnosed. Complete blood count. ESR, urinalysis, blood chemistries, anrinudear antibody test, skin or kidney biopsy. The doctor would prescribe several types of drugs that treats Fred's individual symptoms and needs. Fred also is seeing

144

rheumatologist that specializes in arthritis and other diseases of the joints, bones, and muscles. Neurologist that specializing in disorders of the nervous system. Fred's doctor developed a treatment plan based on Fred's age, health, systems and life style. Fred's treatment plans are tailored to his individual needs. Fred's doctor will reevaluate the plan regularly to ensure that it is as effective as possible. Drugs that decrease inflammation, referred to as non-steroidal, anti-inflammatory drugs (NSAID) are often used.

Paul R. suffers from RHEUMATOID ARTHRITIS

My name is Paul R. and my sister Pam and I have always been good friends. In the 80's I was living in Texas and Pam was still in the Bahamas. My relatives over there told me she was having difficulties like severe pain in her knees, problems walking, reaching, sitting down and doing house hold chores. Her body gets stiff and other parts swell up. Pam was diagnosed with Rheumatoid Arthritis. When I heard she was very sick, I offered to help take care of her. Pam never got along with any of our older brothers, our mother wasn't all that helpful at the time, and our father had already passed away. Pam agreed to come to the United States and live with me, and I became her primary support. My sister arrived in Texas with very few possessions. So I brought her a whole new wardrobe to help her out. She was doing well working for about eighteen months when she had a major relapse. There were some days she couldn't walk, sit or stand or do anything we take for granted every day. When Pm lived with me, I wouldn't let any of our relatives visit us unless they accepted the fact that I'm gay and that Pam has a chronic illness. Pam has changed the lives of everyone in our family. She has given us a wonderful gift. Her arthritis humbled all of us and it has helped everyone in our family become more generous, caring, and sensitive. What is rheumatoid arthritis? Here are the specifics: Managing rheumatoid arthritis (RA) . Successfully begins with learning as much as you can about it. Reading, asking questions and seeking out new information can help you take better control of your own condition. Arthritis is a general term referring to many diseases that can cause pain, stiffness and swelling in joints and other connective tissues. Two common types of arthritis are osteoarthritis (OA) and rheumatoid arthritis (RA). OA, the most common type and the one many people think of when they hear the term "arthritis", that affects the joints. RA, however can affect the whole body and can be progressive and more severe. RA is a disease of the immune system that can result in serious joint damage. In RA, the immune system attacks the body's healthy cells, mistaking them for cells that don't belong. This causes inflammation in the lining and connective tissues of the joints. RA may come on suddenly or appear slowly over time. It's symptoms may include pain, swelling, stiffness in the joints and general tiredness. Fortunately there are medicines that do more than simply treat the symptoms of RA. They may also slow the progressive joint damage of the disease. RA vs. OA- these facts can help clear up some of the confusion between RA and OA. RA: a progressive, damaging disease in which the immune system attacks the body's own joints and other organs. OA- sometimes called "wear and tear" arthritis, resulting fro m age and or repeated intense activity. RA- often affects the entire body and can cause a general feeling of sickness and tiredness. OA- affects only certain joint areas with less effect on your general feeling of well-being. RA generally affects a smaller number of people, but can result in greater changes in the lives of those who have it. More than two million people in the United States have RA. Generally, it affects about twice as many women as men. Although RA can develop in childhood, in most cases it develops between the ages of 25 and 50. RA itself is not inherited.

What can be inherited are the genes that may make someone more likely to develop the disease, including those genes that control your immune system. How fast RA progresses and how severe it differs from person to person. Therefore in diagnosing RA, your physician will need to obtain your individual medical history and conduct a physical examination, including a detailed examination of your joints. Factors such as your current duration of stiffness in the morning, swelling and tenderness of the joints, your ability to move your joints easily, joint heat, and nodules or lumps under your skin are all signs that may indicate you have RA. The pattern of the joints affected may also help your doctor determine whether or not you have RA. RA joints affected in your right hand are usually affected in the left hand as well. There are three powerful reasons why you should seek early diagnosis and treatment for RA. First there's the hidden nature of RA's progressive damage joint. Even after as little as four months, RA can start to damage appears to increase quickly; second there's the fact that joint damage appears to increase quickly. Third, and most important patients who receive early therapy for RA with disease-modifying ant rheumatic drugs also known as DMARDS, may have less pain, swelling, tiredness and morning stiffness as well as slowed joint damage. No treatment is perfect for all people with RA, as the condition is different in every person. But today doctors are more hopeful than ever because of the options they can offer. Currently there are many medicines that can reduce the symptoms of RA. Disease-modifying ant rheumatic drugs (DMARDS) take the process a step further as they may gradually slow the progression of the disease. Recent advances in RA have resulted in new breakthrough medicines. These medicines are bringing new hope to patients and doctors alike. Rheumatologists are prescribing these therapies more and more for people with RA because early therapy has been proven to slow joint damage and may lead to less joint damage and less disability over time. This can mean that people with RA may be able to lead more active lives for a longer period of time. Most people with RA periodic "flare ups" times when the disease is more active and symptoms are more severe, mixed with periods of calm. This can make it difficult to diagnose RA right away. The changing nature, frequency, and seriousness of flare ups also make it easy to understand that many people's moods and emotions are affected as well.

It's perfectly normal to feel anger, fear, and frustration when dealing with this ongoing disease. Dealing with changes in your body and not being able to perform everyday tasks or work at your normal pace can sometimes lead to depression. But once you realize that RA is an ongoing condition and will be a part of your life, you'll have taken the first step toward coping with it successfully. You can help to manage your symptoms and feeling by discussing them with those around you. Create a support system of family, friends, and health care professionals like your doctor, rheumatologist, nurses, physical therapists and others. For many years, exercise was thought to be damaging for people with all kinds of arthritis. Now doctors and therapist know that exercise can actually improve the health and well-being of RA patients by keeping joints moving, music around the joints strong, and the bone and cartilage tissue as strong and healthy as possible. Exercise can also improve your state of mind. Boosting both your self- esteem and your overall sense of well being. Learning how to pace yourself will help you make the most of each day. Saving energy is an important step toward managing your RA, as it helps to make up for the tiredness that often comes along with the disease. Here are some suggestions that may help you feel better and get more done: balance activity with rest, simplify your tasks as much as possible, plan ahead, organize your tasks wisely to avoid tiring out your joints, get help from others. Try linking up with others who are dealing with the same issues. Through articles, RA based web-sites, and support groups, you can share ideas, questions, and success stories with other RA patients. You need to work with your physician. From the start of your RA and throughout its course in your life, your doctor will play an important role in how you understand and manage your condition. More emphasis is now on the mental and social aspects of people with RA as doctors look to treat this disease, which affects day-to-day life. With the breakthrough RA therapies available today, there is greater commitment to relieving every day symptoms and stopping progressive joint damage so you can lead a more fulfilling life. My brother has AIDS and smoked medical marijuana to boost his appetite along with his regular medication. Medical marijuana increased his appetite and relaxed him and eased his pain, so he told his sister Pam, she was reluctant at first. But she trusted her brother so she tried the medical marijuana and almost twenty minutes later she could feel a difference. She was able to relax and her pain was bearable. The medical marijuana also helped with the side effects of her medication.

Mary B suffers from OSTEOPOROSES

Mary B. is a 71 year old grandmother that lives with one of her daughter's whose name is Joan. They live in a small apartment in the city. They have been living together for 7 years since Mary's husband passed away. Joan decided to live with and take care of her mother after her farther passed away. The two women get along fine and understand each other. Of course they have their differences but it's a good match. Mary suffers from Osteoporosis (softening of the bones and increased porosity of the bones) this is mainly found in elderly people. Mary would have to take many types of pain and discomfort medication but one of the pain medications that are not prescribed, that she would request her daughter Joan get for her was marijuana Mary would take marijuana mixed in with green tea every day. She said the green tea mixed with marijuana eased her daily pain and stress. Once a month Joan would buy her mother marijuana from a old school friend. One day Joan had purchased marijuana and was arrested for possession of an illegal substance. She was hand cuffed and made to feel like a common criminal. When Joan was taken to the police station and the police ran her through the computer system she had no record at all. The police person said to her, you have no record so it's evident you're not a criminal, so why did you have marijuana? Joan said, I brought it for my mother. She is in pain due to the illness and asks me to get it for her to help her through the day. The police person said, you know your breaking the law.

Joan said, yes I know. The police person said I understand why you broke the law but you still broke the law and you will have to tell it to a judge on this certain date. Joan was given a date to go to court before a judge. When the day came Joan went before a judge and explains her reasons which the judge understood fully, and was very sympathetic and lenient. The judge dropped all charges on the grounds of Joan being a first time offender. Joan didn't like being made to feel like a criminal being a law abiding person all her life but she understood that some laws are not good and need to be changed. Then I said to Joan, after being arrested, handcuffed, humiliated, made to feel like a common criminal, would you do it again? She looked at me and said, yes, I would do it again, and again, and again. This is my mother and I would do whatever it takes to keep my mother alive and relieve her pain and discomfort. So if it happens again, so be it.

Hope N. suffers from OSTEOARTHRITIS

Hope N. is 55 years old that suffers from Osteoarthritis and has been dealing with it for years now. Hope has always been a active person all her life. She always seems to be traveling and seeing the world and participating in all activities. She probably had excessive stressful use of joints over the years may have caused osteoarthritis in her joints, in her later years. Hope has swelling and stiffness in the joints, particularly after using them. She has loss of flexibility of some joints, back and neck pain. Changes in the weather sometimes causes discomfort in her joints. Hope's knees are greatly affected by osteoarthritis which affects her walking ability. She feels chronic pain when she is walking or just standing in one place. Her hand and feet are also affected as well. Hope is a little over weight and has been doing muscle strengthening exercises on the affected areas which helps the joints. Hope has learned her limitations due to her illness. In Hope's house she has some of the most modern appliances and electronics for convenience of use. That helps make physical application easer. Hope would use a exercise video designed specifically for people with arthritis. The video has gentle routines that in clued stretching, strengthening and fitness exercises.

Throughout the years Hope has been prescribed many different pain medications, stress, and depression medications. She is off the medication that was prescribed to her. Hope had gained more weight, sleeplessness, mood swings, and irritability, and stomach irritation. Hope takes alternative herbal medications for pain, discomfort, swelling. Hope would take marijuana for the pain,, discomfort, depression. Herbs are the basis for many medicines like digitalis, morphine and even aspirin. Scientists are continuing to discover new medicines derived from plants. Herbal preparations are gaining popularity for treating arthritis. Herbs and other plants extracts, are now once again used as alternative pain relievers and inflammation fighters. Marijuana, celery, ginger, devil's claw, cinnamon, avocado, soy extracts, stinging nettle and more. Hope would also take nutritional supplements like vitamins A, C, and E. Salmon oil capsules that have omega-3 fatty acids from cold water Salmon, herring, and mackerel and Aromatherapy (ancient Healers uses oils from plant extracts and resins to promote health and beauty).

GOUT

The gout mainly affects middle age and older men. This disease shows signs of acute arthritis and inflammation of the joints. It will usually start in the feet and knees and begin to increase pain gradually at night time. Thousands of men are affected with this disease on daily bases. People will take different medications and treatments for pain relief. Medical marijuana is taken as one of the pain treatments used by some. Many people that were athletic in their younger lives are now affected with gout as well as people with old injuries. Gout has been around for thousands of years and has had many different treatments from hot compresses to pain killers, to sleeping pills as well as medical marijuana as for pain relief and sleeping aid.

Stiff men syndrome and stiff women syndrome are affected with intermittent tightness, aching, and stiffness of the muscles. Some patients are taking medical marijuana as a relaxer. The gout is recurrent, acute arthritis of the peripheral joints, particularly the great toe. Repeated acute attacks lead to chronic arthritis.

Testimonials - Gout

Sam T. suffers from GOUT

Sam T. is a 55 year old highway road worker who has what is called the Gout, that suddenly first started to affect him when he was 50 years old resulting in intense pain and swelling in a joint of his foot. He also was affected with depression, stress and back pain from a pinched nerve. During the past five years he has had to take off from work many days. There were some days the gout wouldn't let him be able to walk, or go to work. This created more stress and worry about paying bills and keeping his job. Sam's doctor had diagnosed polymyalgia rheumatic arthritis which comes and goes at intervals. Relaxation is required to treat some of these illnesses in conjunction with medicine and medications. Sam would take marijuana for stress, mental depression and pain. He also would take herbal medicine for gout. He would take slippery elm and willow bark for gout. Sam has an uncle and aunt that live upstate on a nice piece of land where they grow corn and other vegetables and herbs. Amongst numerous different types of herbs Sam's aunt grow marijuana for her 85 year old husband and her medical illnesses. Aunt Rose was always know to have what is called a green thumb because she understands how to grow all types of plants. Throughout the years aunt Rose had become a professional cultivator of plants. She would grow marijuana knowing that it was illegal to grow it in her state and yet she continued to grow it for more than thirty years. How she could continue to grow it for so long every year is because it never left the property and was taken by her husband and herself. Their world ended at their property line and the outside world rarely entered into it. If it was not for cable TV and the telephone, when any one went to visit them it was like going back in time with not to many modern features in the house or on the property. They are simple people that believe in a simple way of life that must be working because they are still very active and living long lives.

Tendinitis, Tenosynovitis and Temporomandibular Syndrome

TENDINITIS and TENOSYNOVITIS

Tendinitis and Tenosynovitis are characterized by pain when the joint is moving. Repetitive movements, strain, or excessive exercise may be the causes. Systemic disease may also be the cause like rheumatoid arthritis, gout sclerosis, and infections. Adults over the age of 40 years old and athletes or people with jobs requiring repetitive movement are more likely to acquire tendinitis are taking medical marijuana to treat the pain and discomfort as well as a relaxer.

TEMPOROMANDIBULAR JOINT SYNDROME

Temporomandibular joint syndrome disorder includes congenital and development anomalies like joint disease like arthritis, alkalosis, neoplasm's, or Lupus. The jaw could have been dislocated from a trauma or fracture, teeth clinching or grinding and prolonged stress. Fractures and dislocations produce a shift in the mandible which leads to asymmetric jaw movements, muscle spasms, and pain. Limited jaw movement causes pain. Medical marijuana is taken to relieve stress and pain and to induce relaxation.

Chronic Fatigue and Fibromyalgia

CHRONIC FATIGUE

Chronic Fatigue and Immune Dysfunction Syndrome (CFIDS) also known as the Yuppie Flu. The symptoms are debilitating fatigue, neurologic abnormalities, and persistent symptoms that suggest chronic mononucleosis. It commonly occurs in adults younger than age 45 and its incidence is highest in woman. Some patients are taking marijuana to help with some symptoms such as insomnia or hypersomnia, migratory arthralgia, stress, or depression.

FIBROMYALGIA

Fibromyalgia Syndrome primary symptoms are aching pain concentrated across the neck, lower back, arms, legs, and trunk. Chronic musculoskeletal pain, daily fatigue, and sleep disturbance. Women are affected much more than men, although it can affect all age groups. It may occur as a primary disorder or in association with an underlying disease, such as systemic Lupus Erythematosus, Rheumatoid arthritis, Osteoarthritis, sleep apnea syndromes, and neck trauma. Many patients with this syndrome describe fragmented sleep due to pain or discomfort. Other patients may report feeling tired after a night's sleep. A patient can feel fatigued several hours after awakening and remain so for the remainder of the day. For these sleeping problems, drug therapy is typically used to improve the patient's quality of sleep and pain control. Some patients that have taken these sleeping drugs have improved their sleeping but they had adverse side effects and day time drowsiness. Some of these patients have opted for less sleeping medication, and are taking medical marijuana to help with their sleep and pain and discomfort without any ad versed side effects the next day.

Testimonials - Chronic Fatigue and Fibromyalgia

Tina W. suffered from CHRONIC FATIGUE

Tina W. suffered from Chronic fatigue which led to depression. At first her doctor prescribed amphetamines, which are stimulants, that produce a feeling of increased wakefulness, and energy. These amphetamines temporarily produce a state of normal arousal. Then in a short time Tina became addicted to amphetamines and had to be weaned off of the prescribed amphetamines. Tina is indecisive that's a part of her depression and apprehensive thoughts. She began to loss contact with her friends and relative. When her friends and family would call her, Tina would not return the call back to them. She felt so depressed that she had nothing good or positive to talk with them about and she was avoiding having to talk to others about her depressive feelings. It had gotten more difficult to get up in the morning. Tina would go for treatment of her depression. Her doctor prescribed A prophylactic medication daily in the hope that this would prevent recurrences of this ailment. But the medication was discontinued because Tina didn't like the side effects from it. Her doctor prescribed a different medication that had less side effects. Tina would take marijuana and it would pick up her attitude and she would feel better and be able to function during the day. She would take the marijuana mixed into a herbal tea, that would act like a pick me up drink. It is possible that she has medically unexplained physical symptoms disease. Tina's family would do whatever they could to help her.

Stella S. suffers from FIBROMYALGIA SYNDROME

Stella S. is a 32 year old store manager that is diagnosed with Fibromyalgia syndrome. This ailment is not a type of arthritis but has similarities. With arthritis there is pain in the joints, swelling in the joint, inflammation in the joint. But with Fibromyalgia syndrome it is not the joint itself that is the cause of the pain but the tissues that are near by the joint that is affected. Stella feels the same pain and discomfort as an arthritis patient but there is no swelling of her joints. She feels pain around her knees, hip, neck and elbows. Stella said, that the illness would flare up and then subside and never totally completely disappear. She is unmarried and lives in a small apartment with her two cats and a lot of house plants in flower pots on all the window sills in the apartment. She is the type of person known as what's called a loner. She has very few friends if any and prefers to live alone with her pets. To hear Stella tell how non eventful her life is and seemingly boring to me, she loved it that way. She loved being alone, just her cats and plants was all she wants, that makes her happy. I got the impression that Stella probably had some traumatic experiences with people in her past.

When Stella was diagnosed with Fibromyalgia she said, the doctor had good news and some bad news as well. The good news was that the illness was not progressive, disabling or life threatening. The bad news was that she would have it for the rest of her life. As time moved on Stella learned how to deal with the pain and continue to work on her job. She said that she tried many pain killers, medicines and medications and she said that she still prefers to take marijuana to help her in those times she has painful moments. She also said, outside of taking marijuana for pain it's a good sleep aid. Stella said, that she buys it from a friend on her job and sometimes grows marijuana in her apartment in small amounts. Of course when she tries to grow it in her apartment in flower pots, . The plants never matured enough to produce a high THC content. Never the less she still tries to grow it every year and gets better and better every year. Stella may have a boring life but it's what she wants to do with it and if that's what makes her happy then it's alright.

Sciatica

There have been a few reports stating that many people that are suffering from Sciatica pain attacks are taking medical marijuana, in addition to other pain killers. Some of these people have had back surgery due to a defective intervertebral disk and still take medical marijuana as pain management. People that have Sciatica know how survey the pain is that goes down their leg through the sciatic nerve. Other pain treatment drugs are morphine or Demerol for a short period of time.

Testimonials - Scoliosis and Sciatica

Jennifer S. suffers from SCIATICA PAIN

Jennifer S. is a 32 year old hair stylist that suffers from Sciatica pain due to having Scoliosis and from a recent car accident in which she received a back injury. Jennifer's husband Kevin had helped her through the long ordeal after the car accident that Jennifer was in. After the accident so many things in her life had changed. She had a slow and lengthy recovery which was painful. After a year Jennifer was not 100 per cent and may never be again but she would learn to live with it. She still had Sciatica back pain and leg pain frequently. Having tried numerous different types of pain killers and medications in which very little would help outside of a needle shot of heavy duty narcotics. Jennifer chose to opt for a combination of medications that to function during a normal day's activities. One of the medications was medical marijuana to help deal with having the back pain and as a pick me up medication. Some of Jennifer's doctors suggested that corrective spinal surgery might help or there is a possibility that she might be paralyzed after the spinal surgery. For Jennifer the words (might help) was not enough for her to take the chance of the possibility of becoming paralyzed. Jennifer required a guarantee that she would not become paralyzed if she had such a intricate operation on her back so she opted not to have the operation and seek other means of pain relief. She believed the medical technology was not yet advanced enough to guarantee her not becoming paralyzed. So until there were more of a likelihood of achievement, she would wait until then.

Jennifer is learning how to be less active and more careful with her body movement so as to not aggravate her back condition. She would have to learn how to watch her diet and eat the right foods. She went for canceling with a dietician and food expert. The dietician made suggestions of different foods for her needs and condition. Due to her job she has a limited time to take care of all the things that she has to do during the course of a day. Jennifer would continue to take marijuana in herbal tea to help her appetite and help her pain management. Her husband Kevin would get her the marijuana knowing that it was against the laws in his state but in his mind if marijuana was helping his wife then he had no choice but to help her in any way he could. He realized that sometimes we have to do some things for loved ones that we don't wish to do. But we will do whatever it takes to help that loved one.

Allen D. suffers from SCIATICA PAIN

Allen D. suffers from intermittent and sometimes constant Sciatica back pain at the age of 37. Having had to deal with this physical problem for years even had back surgery at one time. Allan said that at times the pain would be so intense that it would be unbearable and painful to move and cause great pain. The pain would disable him to a degree where he could not go to work. He would go back and forth to the doctors for a shot of heavy duty pain medication. During one of his trips in the doctor's office he met a woman with a similar problem. Her name is Matilda. She is a 28 year old art designer that suffers from sciatica back pain due to a car accident several years prior. Allan and Matilda saw that they have more in common than they thought. They began to see each other and trade information about how to deal with their sciatica back pain. They would still take the doctors prescribed pain medications but much less. Matilda prefers to take medical marijuana along with other pain medication as she has been doing for the last several years. She had went through a gauntlet of testing pain killers and medication and seem to settle with certain pain tablets and marijuana as a mental relaxer. Being and art designer she spends a lot of time at her computer which aggravated her sciatica pain that would run down her back to one of her legs that would affect her walking ability. Allan and Matilda would see each other just on the weekends were they like to go to different places. Matilda's parents own a summer house in the country just two hour's drive from the city where they live. Matilda and Allan made a date to spend a quiet week end at Matilda's parents country house. They both looked forward to the upcoming week end so the Friday before they were to go, they would check to make sure they had everything they needed for their week end. Like food, changes of clothes and other things. Matilda would go up to her parents country house at least once or twice a month to get away from the hustle and bustle of the city. While she would be at the country house she would tend her garden and the flowers on the property. She would bring with her plant food, fertilizers, and starter plants. Matilda had quite a green thumb when it came to botany of plants of all types. Having learned throughout the years what was best for the growth of flowers, vegetables and herbs. For her this was a hobby that she loves to do. She had taken botany classes in school and was at the top of her class in this course. She also studied how to grow plants in extreme environments for the best results. Her hobby of botany has a therapeutically affect on Matilda which was relaxing for her. But at times was hard physical work especially if a person has sciatica back pain.

When they arrived at the country house and began to unpack heir things, Allan came across he plant food which seemed so out of place to him. Allan asked Matilda about the plant food. Matilda hesitated for a minute and said, let me show you why I brought the plant food with us. She took Alan by the hand and walk with him outside to the back of the house and showed him that she had a garden in the back. Where she grows vegetables, flowers and different herbs. One of them was marijuana that she said she would take to help her sciatica back pain. When Allan saw it he was surprised but he understood. Allan said, to Matilda that this answers a lot of questions like he always wonder where and how she would buy marijuana when in reality she was growing it. Matilda had been growing marijuana for her personal us for several years. Every year she grows just enough for herself and to last until the next year and then she repeats the process. By doing his she wouldn't have to buy it or deal with dealers. She kept this to herself knowing it was not legal in her state to grow. Matilda made the choice to grow marijuana because she felt it was one of the pain medications that gave her relief as well as a mental boost or pick me up. They savored every minute of there week end together not wanting it to end and it would be Monday morning the beginning of another week again. As time moved on Allan would take medical marijuana to give himself pain relief along with other medications. Allan and Matilda soon fell in love and would spend many weekends together, they soon got married. As a wedding gift Matilda's parents gave her the country house and property. They moved there and Matilda would work from home and Allan would commute to work. Matilda found that she did her best art design work from the privacy of her home. She still had sciatica pain but not as severe as in the past. They still see their doctors and therapy sessions and they would have more progress each time. Allan and Matilda would take the marijuana only when their pain was intense for relief. Matilda learned how to conceal the marijuana plants with other plants and change its physical appearance to not grow tall. She was such a good botanist that she could graft a marijuana plant with another type of herb to look totally different from the original marijuana plant and have the same THC content as a marijuana plant. This was not very easy to do and had to be done perfectly in order to work but Matilda could do it, and every time. After a while the marijuana plants look nothing like what a marijuana plant normally looks like.

LUPUS

Systemic Erythematosus (Lupus) is a type of immune system disorder known as an autoimmune disease. In autoimmune diseases the body harms its own healthy cells and tissues. This leads to inflammation and damage of various body tissues. Lupus can affect many parts of body, including the joints, skin, kidneys, heart, lungs, blood vessels, and brain. Although people with the disease may have many different symptoms, some of the most common ones include extreme fatigue, painful or swollen joints, arthritis, unexplained fever, skin rashes, and kidney problems. Lupus is also known as a rheumatic disease. The rheumatic diseases are a group of disorders that cause aches, pain, and stiffness in the joints, muscles, and bones. Symptoms of Lupus can be controlled with appropriate treatment and most people with the disease can lead active, healthy lives. At present there is no cure for Lupus. However, the symptoms of Lupus can be controlled with appropriate treatment. Lupus is characterized by periods of illness, called flares, and periods of wellness, or remission. Understanding how to prevent flares and how to treat them when they do occur helps people with Lupus maintain better health. Intense research is underway and scientists funded by the NH are continuing to make great strides in understanding the disease, which ultimately may lead to a cure. Two of the questions researchers are studying are who gets Lupus and why. We know that many more woman then men have b Lupus. Lupus is three times more common in black woman than in white woman and is also more common in woman of Hispanic, Asian, and Native American Indians. In addition, Lupus can run in families, but the risk that a child or a brother or sister of a patient also will have Lupus is still quite low. It is difficult to estimate how many people in the United States have the disease because its symptoms very widely and its onset is often hard to pinpoint. Lupus is not infectious and mainly affects woman.

Lupus is an autoimmune disease which is chronic and causes inflammation of various parts of the body. The immune system protects the body against bacteria, foreign materials, and viruses. In autoimmune disease like Lupus, the immune system loses its ability to tell the difference between foreign substances and its own cells and tissues. The immune system then makes antibodies directed against its self. The symptoms come and go and mimic many other illnesses. Some symptoms of Lupus are joint swelling, muscle pain, rashes, fevers, hair loss, appetite loss, sores, painful sensitivity of the fingers, Lupus is more prevalent than AIDS, Sickle Cell Anemia, Cystic Fibrosis, and Multiple Sclerosis, combined. Lupus affects 1 out of every 185 people and strikes adult woman 15 times more frequently than men. Medical marijuana is taken to help with pain and discomfort and as a appetite inducer. Although Lupus ranges from mild to life threatening, the majority of cases can be controlled with proper treatment. While medical science has not yet developed a method for curing Lupus. New research brings increased hope each year.

Mary D. suffers from LUPUS

There is another story about a woman called Mary D., at the age of 45 years old she was diagnose with a life threatening disease called Lupus. Lupus is a disease causes the body to produce to many antibodies or proteins. There are various forms of lupus. Some forms of lupus may show symptoms of affecting the kidneys, lungs, nervous system and the joints of the body. Low white blood cells and red blood cells and abnormalities of blood antibodies caused by the disease. Mary is suffering with systemic lupus. How one develops this disease is unknown. Her symptoms are swollen joints, pain, achiness, swollen glands, lack of energy. Her pain and discomfort can be unbearable at times and after going to doctors for over a year and feeling like a Ginny pig. At times she was prescribed cancer fighting drugs as well as steroids and other test drugs. She did not know whether or not the test drugs were the cause of her kidney damage or derived from systemic lupus disease. Difficulty sleeping, joint pain, swelling, stiffness, muscle pain and stress are just a few ailments she suffers from. She had been prescribed numerous amounts of drugs to combat theses ailments but she did not like some of these drugs that make her to sleepy or groggy to a point where she could not deal with life's daily matters. Mary realized that she needed help from any and all. She began to try alterative medications such as herbal and vitamins as well as medical marijuana. She found that the marijuana helps with dealing with the stress of lupus decrease. Marijuana had a combing effect on her mental condition and elevated stress without the heavy drug feeling in her system. Medical marijuana can be prescribed with a prescription by a doctor but most do not. Those doctors that do prescribe medical marijuana do so in pill form which is not the same as taking it in organic form. When taking marijuana in pill form the patient can't regulate the amount of dosage intake. When taking marijuana in smoke form the patient can regulate the intake amount as needed. Mary realized that it was against most state laws to grow marijuana but she also realized that the times we live in that all laws are not infallible and laws change in time. Her time is now and fleeting away so she decided to grow marijuana in her garden with the other plants. Being that Mary is a none smoker she prefers to ingest marijuana mixed in with herbal teas and foods. Mary became a cultivator out of necessity to ease the ailments and continue her life. Her mental state was more optimistic and her stress levels went down. She doesn't like the idea of breaking the state laws but she was looking at the bigger picture.

Testimonials - Multiple Disorders

Marie L. suffers from MULTIPLE ILLNESSES

Marie L. is a 38 year old mother of a 8 year old child. Marie is suffering from a combination of illnesses one of which is Lupus disease, another is depression which causes stress. Marie is a single parent that is not working due to the Lupus disease. She is collecting child support for her child whose name is May and she also is collecting Social Security disability payments for having ADD disorder. Marie's illness prevents her from working a 9 to 5 job. With child support payments and her disability payments Marie is able to maintain a stable home for May and herself in a two bedroom apartment. By no means is she what's called well off financially but manages to make ends meet.

No one really knows how, where or why a person acquires Lupus whether it is due to a chemical imbalance or change in one's body due to aging or a mental factor. Lupus is not transmittable or infectious to others but it can be as devastating as the AIDS disease. Marie has basically an upbeat personality except when she has bouts of depression which can trigger her stress and sometimes the reverse. After Marie found out that she had Lupus some of her greatest worries was how is she going to provide for herself and her child and if something had happened to her. Who would take care of May? Fortunately Marie does have some one that she can count on. His name is Phillip who has been Marie's boyfriend for six years. Phillip was always there in times of need for Marie. Even though Phillip did not live with Marie, he was the only father May ever knew and treated her as if she was his own biological child. Marie realized that Phillip had always been there to cover her and May's best interest. Being that Marie had a very aggressive type of Lupus which drained her energy, caused swelling in different areas of her body at different times. One day the swelling may be in a knee or elbow, hand or other part of her body. The swelling is only one aspect of the Lupus disease there are many more which could lead to premature death. Marie would take prescribed drugs and medications to combat the effects of the Lupus disease but she would prefer to take medical marijuana for her depression and stress which was provided for her by Phillip who would take it to relax. Marie would make Phillip as her legal guardian and to care for May if something should ever happen to her. It had been planned that Phillip and his parents would take care of and raise May if anything happened to her mother. Marie and Phillip would have to do their best to see that this doesn't happen. By fighting this disease and any mental problems.

Catherine C. is affected by MULTIPLE ILLNESSES

Some people are affected with multiple illnesses like a middle age woman named Catherine C. Catherine who is a famous movie star and well known. She had been diagnosed with fibrocystic breast disease and had recently had a subcutaneous mastectomy. She also was affected with carpel tunnel syndrome. After she had the mastectomy she would worry about being in sexual situations with men for fear of not appearing like a complete woman. Catherine also worried about getting acting roles if the movie companies find out that she has had a mastectomy. Being a famous actress it is hard to have any privacy or a life of an average person. Most actresses lives are open books for all to see. But sometimes we have no choice but to change one's life style. Catherine being a versatile person would have to learn to adapt to her situation. She would now be more selective in choosing the acting roles she was offered. She became a lot less active in romantic interludes. Catherine was taking pain medicines to help with the carpal tunnel syndrome in her hands that gave her sometimes great discomfort. She also found out that marijuana is a mild relaxer that calms her nerves. Catherine knew that it is illegal to have marijuana in her state so she stopped taking marijuana for several months and would take other medicines that she said were ineffective. So she went back to taking marijuana in the evenings for relief. She would soon become an advocate for the use of marijuana for the treatment of medical illnesses. Catherine became a voice for the state legalization of marijuana for medical use. She would become a leader in her state for the changing of the laws pertaining to medical marijuana.

Elaine H. suffers from CRAMPS

Elaine H. is a 45 year old business women that suffers from cramps. She has always seem to suffer from cramps right after puberty. Some women have a light phase when there cramps come, where as some other women have a heavy cramp cycle time. The ones that have a heavy cramp cycle have pain, stress, weakness, and fatigue. This happens to many women all over the world. Whereas the women that have a light cramp cycle don't have half the problems of the heavy cramp cycle type of women. Elaine has dealt with this most of her life and has learned how to deal with it. She makes sure that she eats healthy foods to make sure her body is prepared for next month's cycle. After having to deal with heavy cramps for many years Elaine has it down to a science of treatment. As one of her treatments is the use of medical marijuana as a pain and stress reliever as well as stomach reliever. Elaine has been taking medical marijuana for many years with no problem with it in conjunction with other medications or it being habit forming. Throughout the years she has taken medical marijuana and she says that she will continue to take medical marijuana in the future, because it helps her during her cramp cycle. Elaine said, she knows she is breaking the State laws, and has been breaking the law for years. She said that she would rather not break the law, but the law needs to be changed pertaining to medical marijuana in most States to help people in need of their illnesses. Then she turned and said, by the way, you are not using my real name, right? Right.

Other herbs taken are Melissa officlnalis, Artemisia vulgaris, bayberry {Myrica cerifera}. Weight loss cannabinoid: Acomplia also known as Rimonabant- for the treatment of obesity was recently legalized with prescription by the regulatory authorities in Europe. This is the first cannabinoid antagonist on the market in pill form. Acomplia blocks the natural binding of endogenous cannabinoids and THC. This causes a lack of appetite and weight loss. It will be available in the United States in the near future if it passes the FDA tests. I have no comment on it at this time, let's wait and see.

Kathrin S. suffers from SEVERAL ILLNESSES

Kathrin S. suffers from several illnesses. Arthritis, stiff woman's syndrome, elevated stress, glaucoma. Kathrin is 58 years old but she looks like she is 48 years old and she said, she sometimes feels like she is 98 years old due to the pain and discomfort. Kathrin is home bound and collects Social Security disability payments. She also is a grandmother of a 6 year old boy and a 7 year old girl. Kathrin takes care of the children 5 days a week, for three hours a day until her daughter gets off from work and comes to take the children home. Kathrin would have to walk two blocks to the school bus stop to escort the children to her house and baby sit until their mother came to pick them up. It use to be that it was very painful for Kathrin to walk the two blocks to the bus stop and then two blocks back to her house. The arthritis has affected her legs which makes walking very painful. She tries not to show any pain around the children so they don't worry about her. She use to be stressed out over not being able to keep up with the children when in the house due to her lack of mobility. The arthritis feet, knees and hands mainly. Kathrin had a operation on her eyes that had helped her with the glaucoma illness. She takes different medications that do not conflict with each other. She also takes medical marijuana in herbal teas twice a day. Once in the midday and one cup in the evening. She said that she knew that medical marijuana was not yet legalized in her State yet but the pain and discomfort and lack of mobility was too much to bear. She said that she has tried everything and medical marijuana in tea relieves some pain and discomfort as well as help her sleep at night and increase her appetite. Kathrin said, she did a little test to see if the marijuana was having these effects by stop taking the herbal tea mix for one week. She found that she had more pain and discomfort, sleepless nights that caused stress and lack of appetite for that week. She continued to take the medical marijuana in herbal tea twice a day and manage to baby sit her grand children after school. Kathrin didn't say where she got the medical marijuana and I didn't ask. Most people will get marijuana from a friend or relative and take it for their particular illness. For people like Kathrin that do not smoke at all, they will take it in foods or liquids like tea. Kathrin mixes marijuana with mint leaves, and regular tea. The tea mix, does not contract with the other pain medication she has to take on a daily basis.

Mr. and Mrs. Lee use herbs to help their illnesses

For thousands of years Asia herbal healers have been prescribing marijuana for treatment. In China the Chinese herbal healers have it down to a fine art of accuracy in prescribing the correct herbal medicine for specific illnesses. As well in Myanmar, Thailand, Vietnam, and India. An elderly couple named Wo and Mayling Lee of Nanning China lived on their farm raising chickens and growing vegetables. It came to light that Mr. Lee had arthritis in his hands which prevented him from maintaining his farm work. After trying different doctors and medications with no positive results. Mrs. Lee began to do more work around the farm to take up the slack for her husband but that soon began to take its toll on her. The stress and pressure of her husband's illness and extra work drove her into depression. Mrs. Lee was told by a local herbal healer to take Green tea and marijuana in the late afternoons which was having a positive effect on her stress and depression. It helped her cope with her situation. Mr. Lee would smoke the marijuana in a handmade pipe saying that it helped the discomfort in his hands. In Vietnam the hemp plants which are marijuana is used for many different purposes from rope, clothes, brooms, baskets, and medicine combinations. In most of the villages the people relied on what they grow and utilizing what their environment offers. Marijuana has been used all over the world for thousands of years for medical use.

ALZHEIMER'S DISEASE

Alzheimer's disease is also known as primary degenerative dementia. People that suffer from this have mild to moderate dementia. As dementia progressed the patient mind becomes more degenerative. Medical Marijuana is taken for several reasons, to help the patient's mood and as an antidepressant to treat depression. Research has found that the THC in marijuana inhibits the enzyme responsible for the aggregation of amyloidal plaque. The THC in marijuana and its analogues provide an improved therapeutic option for Alzheimer's disease by simultaneously treating both the progression of the disease and the symptoms. Tests are still being done to prove that medical marijuana causes improvement in memory and a reduction in inflammation.

Testimonials - Alzheimer's Disease

Grand Pa is suffering from ALZHEIMER'S DISEASE

Grand Pa is suffering from Alzheimer's disease at the age of 88. Grand Pa lives with one of his son's named Stanly that takes care of him. Stanley's wife and three children also help take care of Grand Pa and keep an eye on him due to the fact that Grand Pa would forget many things at times, like people's names, locations of places he had been in previously. When Grand Pa was younger he was very outgoing and totally independent in everything he did. From building his own electronics company out of nothing to a multi-million dollar firm that ships electronics all over the world. The electronics company is now controlled by a board of directors for the last 8 years after Grand Pa had retired from the company. These days Grand Pa can't even remember what he had for dinner last night or how to do the little thing that one normally does during the cores of a regular day. Like wash up in the morning or dressing properly. He doesn't remember people from his past or their faces or names. Before the disease started to progress Grand Pa would get frustrated about not being able to remember certain important personal memories and would start to cry. It was very hard watching him deter ate a little more every day. One day Stanley's oldest son was to be married and was having a party at the house in the basement recreation area.

Stanley's son is called Stan Jr. and had four of his friends over for the party and his four friends hired two woman to put on a dance show and show special attention to the groom. When the party was starting to cook about midnight Grand Pa came down the stairs to see where the loud music was coming from, having forgotten that his grandson Stan Jr. was getting married. Some one of the girls said who is that? Stan said oh that's my Grand farther, I'll take him back up stairs to his room. The same girl said no don't take him away please let him stay for a while, he might have a good time too. Stan replied alright he can stay for a little while. Stan said, that his Grand farther has Alzheimer's disease and doesn't talk much. Stan's friends where drinking alcohol and passing a joint around to each other and the joint made its way around to Grand Pa. Stan said no don't give the joint to Grand Pa, it might mess him up more than he already is. One of the girls said to Stan, you are treating your Grand farther like he is a child and he does not look like he's totally out of it. Give him the joint and see what he does with it. They past the joint to Grand Pa and he took two big drags off of the joint and held the smoke in for some time and a smile came over his face.

One of the woman said, see Grand Pa likes it and she sat on Grand Pa's lap and he smiled even more. The woman said, see he even likes this more and then she got up laughing. Then out of the clear blue sky Grand Pa said, it's been a very long time since I had a beautiful young woman sit on my lap and it felt good. Stan's mouth drop open in shock hearing his Grand farther speak a whole sentence that made sense. The woman said to Stan, I thought you said that your grandfather couldn't speak? Stan replied, he can't speak and the woman said, well he can speak now jokingly. Grand Pa got up from the chair and turned and said, nice to meet you all and thank you for a good time. He then went up the stairs to bed. The next day Stan told his father Stanly what had happen at the party and that Grand Pa had spoke to them and came out of his usual catatonic state that he is always in. At first Stanly didn't believe what his son was saying because Grand Pa hasn't spoken a full sentence in two years. Stanly would have to see if the marijuana did help his farther to remember anything and come out of the catatonic state he was in. Stanly planned to do this the next day which was Saturday. Stanly was off from work and plan to cook outside on the back yard barbeque gill, Saturday afternoon. This particular day so happen that everyone that lives in the house was out except Stanly, Stan Jr. and Grand Pa. Stanly cooked a few steaks and ears of corn for Grand Pa and himself. After Stanly and Grand Pa had eaten Stanly lit a joint of marijuana and took a little drag from it and past the joint to Grand Pa. Grand Pa took one drag and then another and then another. Stanly said dad, do you remember anything? His father gave no reply. Stanly said dad, do you remember mother, your wife? Once again he gave no response. Stanly thought to himself, saying, I knew it wasn't going to work and got up and started to walk to the back door. When he heard a voice say, Stanly tell your mother to bring out my coat. I'm cold. Stanly quickly turned around with a joyous look on his face of surprise and said, dad you remember mother and me and your talking again. Then Grand Pa said, next time son you cook me corn make sure you cut the kernels off the stork to make it easier on my benchers, and tenderize my steak which makes it a little easier for me to chew. Stanly replied, why yes dad with a smile. Then Grand Pa fell back into, a catatonic state. Stanly had told his wife about the Grand Pa test and what had happen. Stanly said that the marijuana did help his farther remember a few things and speak a few words. Even though Grand Pa's wife had passed away many years ago, at least he had remember he had a wife and that I'm still his son. The marijuana seem to affect bits and pieces of Grand Pa's memory almost as if, it were a light being turn on and then off. Stanly felt that the marijuana would help save or regain Grand Pa's memory but didn't like the idea of having to buy an illegal drug that helps his dad's memory. Stanly felt that he would have to do whatever it takes to help his father in his last years be comfortable.

Charlotte B. suffers from AMYOTROPHIC LATERAL SCLEROSIS

Charlotte B. suffers from Amyotrophic Lateral Sclerosis (ALS). The most command name for this disease is Lou Gehrig's Disease. At the age of 47 ALS attacked her legs with paralysis of her leg muscles. The diseases attack was swift and decisive. It seemed to happen overnight, one day Charlotte was walking, running and dancing and the next day she was in a wheel chair. Being in a wheel chair was very difficult for her after having been very active in her life. Charlotte was the type of person that has traveled all over the world, from one end to the other. When she was younger, she was a over sea plane stewardess, and has been traveling ever since. And now she was like a fish out of water. She went from doctor to doctor and the answer was still the same. There's nothing we can do. For whatever reason the disease had slowed it's progression to only effecting half her body, the lower part. She was told that the paralysis of her leg muscles was permanent, but she's not the type to give up and lay down and die. She is a fighter and searched out alternative medicines.

She went to a healer that used hands on healing, self hypnotism, and recommended certain herbal medicines including marijuana in teas or smoked. In about a week Charlotte saw a little progress, she was able to move her big toe, when this happen she felt joy, happiness, relieve and renew hope. Charlotte knew she could beat this disease with the weapons she has now. She would continue to see the healer and take the herbal medicines recommended. Slowly she would exercise her toes and then feet and legs. She would have a regiment of muscle strengthening exercises to help her walk again. After several months, Charlotte was walking without the use of a cane or walker. She stopped seeing the healer but keep his phone number just in case she has a (ALS) relapse. She would continue to take the recommend herbal medicines including marijuana.

Brian S. suffers from MULTIPLE SCLEROSIS

Brian S. is a 42 year old stock broker that was diagnosed with Multiple Sclerosis in its early stages. Brian is married with two children in college. Before he was diagnosed with M.S. he was experiencing muscle pain, weakness, cramps, ataxia motor. At times he would experience vertigo when Brian would simply be walking down the street. He had a lack of deep sensibility that cause lack of equilibrium in standing. He had rhizotomy posterior surgery done to relieve unresponsive spasms. He was prescribed muscle relaxants for spasticity and corticosteroids for acute attacks, and some test drugs. He would work from home when he was not feeling well enough to go into the stock office. His wife would help him when the spasm attacks were bad. Brian would take marijuana with other medications to ease his pain and discomfort. He has constantly stated that marijuana is one of the only medications that helps him with his illness. In the state that Brian lives there is no program or laws pertaining to the legalization of medical marijuana so it is not available as a prescription medication. Brian would purchase it illegally from a friend. Brian started a petition drive for the legalization for medical marijuana in his state with thousands of signatures from people with different illnesses of all types that needed medical marijuana. Times are changing and soon medical marijuana will be legal for medical use by prescription in Brian's state. Aunt Rose was expert with each plant and it's best way of cultivation. With marijuana she would grow it like a bonsai plant, in doing so the plants did not look like the typical tall marijuana stalk but like a shrub bush which are hard to detect. This is just one of many plants that aunt Rose cultivated to promote longer and better health. Sam would visit his uncle and aunt once a month and stay the week end to help out around the properties with maintenance like cutting the bushes and grass. Aunt Rose would make herbal tea and different meals that she incorporated marijuana with other herbs in meals. Sam preferred to smoke the marijuana out of a small pipe. To look at Sam's uncle Eddy and aunt Rose you see a white haired elderly man and woman that look much younger than they really are. Neither one of them have seemed to slowed down physically or mentally. It seemed as if time had stood still or slowed down for this couple or could it be that there life style was aiding in there longevity. The property was five acres with a stream running through it with woods and a meadow and a two hundred year old colonel house. The four seasons always seemed to come on queue with the calendar, hot green summers, cool orange fall, cold white winters and then starts all over again with yellow warmth of the sun of spring This couple knows how to live with the land and sessions. The land has a mystical air about it as if your entering a peaceful content place which requires a lot of hard work.

Drug and Alcohol Addiction

DRUG ADDICTION

The sustained use of many kinds of drugs causes adaptations within the body that tend to lessen the drug's original effects over time, a phenomenon known as drug tolerance. At this point, one is said to also have a physical dependency on the given chemical. This is the stage that withdrawal may be experienced upon discontinuation. Some of these symptoms are generally the opposite of the drug's direct effect on the body. Depending on the length of time a drug takes to leave the bloodstream elimination half-life, withdrawal symptoms can appear within a few hours to several days after discontinuation and may also occur in the form of cravings. A craving is the strong desire to obtain, and use a drug or other substance similar to other cravings one might experience for food and hunger.

ALCOHOL ADDICTION

Alcoholism is a broad term for problems with alcohol, and is generally used to mean compulsive and uncontrolled consumption of alcoholic beverages, usually to the detriment of the drinker's health, personal relationships, and social standing. It is medically considered a disease, specifically an addictive illness, and in psychiatry several other terms are used, specifically "alcohol abuse" and "alcohol dependence," which have slightly different definitions. Excessive use of alcohol leads to tolerance, physical dependence, and an alcohol withdrawal syndrome. The withdrawal syndrome is largely due to the central nervous system being in a hyper-excitable state. The withdrawal syndrome can include seizures and delirium tremens and may lead to excito-neurotoxicity.

Many former alcoholics are taking marijuana. A survey was taken and found that a large number of former alcoholics are taking marijuana along with a lot of coffee drinking and cigarette smoking to relax and ease the urges of the previous alcohol addiction. Adult ADD is a disorder that requires medicine like adder all, and Ritalin that when are taken to check the disorder one of the side effects is loss of appetite. Marijuana is used to increase the patients appetite so that the patient can maintain good nutrition and body weight. Adult ADD requires the same type of medicine that's used to treat ADD so it has the same side effects which is the loss of appetite and marijuana is used to increase the patients appetite. Some other herbal medicines used to treat alcoholics are Artichoke for liver protection, Kava, SAMe, St. Johns Wort, Cordyceps.

Testimonials - Drug and Alcohol Addiction

Harry S. suffers from a FORMER CRACK ADDICTION

Harry S. is a 35 year old that is an X-crack addict that is trying to get his life back. Harry had been a crack and cocaine addict for 10 years until he went to get help and rehabilitation from his crack addiction. He signed himself into a rehabilitation clinic for 2 months which took a lot of courage on Harry's part, but he knew that he needed help to get rid of the addiction. Once Harry completed the detox program and went home he knew, he would have to not associate with the old crowd of friends that were still doing crack and cocaine. He would, as they say, cut the old crowd loose. He would have to make new friends, new friends that are not into crack and cocaine. Harry got a job as a stock man and in a few months he was doing well. One day as he was going to work he happened to see coming toward him was a crack addict friend from Harry's past. Harry thought to himself, it's too late to avoid contact with the old friend, so might as well say, hello. It was obvious that the old friend was still using crack from his appearance, looking dirty and malnourished. The old friend said, Harry, long time, no see. You look good, where have you been hanging out all this time? Harry said, I've been around. The old friend said to Harry, I'm going to score, you want to come?

Harry said, no, no thanks I'm on my way to work now, maybe some other time. Harry thought to himself, I'm never going back to that old life and old habits. As Harry turned to walk away the old friend said, you have a job? As if the friend was surprised that Harry could hold a job. Maybe the old Harry couldn't hold a job but the new Harry can. Harry still and maybe always have the urge every now and then for crack but he wouldn't go for it. What he would do instead was to smoke marijuana and that would decrease his urges for crack and he would not be seduced by crack urges. The marijuana not only would decrease his urges for crack but also would increase his appetite thus eating more food and becoming healthier all round. Harry would always remember that day he ran into the crack addicted friend and how bad the friend looked. Harry made himself a promise, not to go down that path ever again.

Jesse W. suffers from a FORMER ALCOHOL ADDICTION

Jesse W. is a 37 year old x-alcoholic that has been clean from alcohol for four years without a drink. About 95% of Jesse's old friends drink some kind of alcohol so it was difficult for Jesse to socialize with them. When he was around them, they would offer him a drink and it was hard for him to refuse, but he did. And when he refused he was made to feel like an outsider by not drinking with them. After a while Jesse's old friends stopped calling him to hang out and party (go out drinking). Whenever Jesse wanted a drink of alcohol, he would smoke some marijuana to relax the stress of wanting a drink. Jesse felt like an outsider with some of his old friends. He would deal with it by not drinking with them. Jesse would go home after work, smoke some marijuana, and relax and think to himself, I'm better off without friends like that any way. I'll make new friends that aren't drinkers. Jesse went to a few places where there is non-alcoholic drinks served. It didn't take long before Jesse had some new non alcoholic drinking friends, and he met new women to. Some of Jesse's new friends are x-alcoholic's as well. They all seem to take something to ease the stress of each day without a drink. Some will drink a lot of hot coffee and smoke cigarettes. Others will eat more food, for Jesse and several others they will take marijuana to ease their stress or depression. One day Jesse got a phone call from one of his old drinking friends that informed Jesse that there had been a tragic car accident. One of Jesse's drinking, hang out buddies was killed in a car accident, due to driving under the influence of alcohol. Jesse felt bad and wondered what he could have done to prevent it from happening. Jesse realized that he would have probably been killed to because the friend that died would always pick up Jesse and drive to where the other friends were. Jesse had gone to that friend's funeral to show respect and say good bye to an old friend. Jesse would never forget that old friend and dedicate himself to helping the other hang out drinking buddies stop their alcohol abuse.

PERSONALITY NEUROSIS DISORDER

There are many walking right now with personality neurosis disorder and do not even know they have a disorder. Personality neurosis is a disorder of the thought processes not do to a physical disease but probably due to some unresolved mental internal conflicts which make for an uneasy adjustment to life. There are many types of neurosis like anxiety, phobic, obsessive compulsive, hysteria, reactive, depression. The everyday pressers and problems ad to mental fatigue, worry, distress. Mood Swings: Everyone has them and they affect everyone differently. Mood Swings are controlled by the combination of our thoughts and feelings which could put us in a good mood or a bad mood.

Most of us experience these mood swings and there different degrees in between feeling happy or feeling sad. Some people cannot simply think their way out of a bad mood which could stay with them for some time or sad mood or sad mood which could last for some time. These people would take medical marijuana instead of a drink of alcohol or heavy drugs. Medical marijuana seems to relax them as well as put them in a happier and more optimistic frame of mind. It seems to change ones ideas and thought alternatives.

Other herbal medicines that are used to treat these disorders are Asian Ginseng, Gortu Kola, St. Johns Wort, Mother Wort.

Testimonials - Neurasthenia

Janet K. suffers from NEURASTHENIA

Janet K. is a 57 year old woman that suffers from Neurasthenia which is a disease commonly following depression that displays various symptoms of types of organic diseases without the existence of any organic diseases sufficient to justify the complaints of Janet K.,. In other words the Doctors can't find anything physically wrong with her to cause her complaints. Janet had been grieving over the death of her farther that passed away the previous year at the age of 90 years. Janet's husband Martin noticed almost immediately the change in his wife as far as mental and physically. Janet was very close with her farther and was hurt if not devastated after his passing and had heavy depression. Janet would start to complain of weakness, headaches, poor sleeping, aches, pain and exhaustion. In the house where Martin and Janet have been living in for over 30 years there are three stair cases. All of a sudden lately Janet becomes easily exhausted when even walking up just one stair case from the first floor to the second floor of the house. Janet would walk up the stairs and by the time she got to the top step she would have to sit down to take a rest. Martin took Janet from Doctor to Doctor and specialist to specialist and still nothing physical was found. After a while it was believed that her problems were psychological due to the stress of losing her father. As time moved on Janet got progressively worse with the development other new symptoms like vertigo and photophobia, pain. All of these things began to make her irritable and complain about everything. Her husband Martin very understood about why she would complain and seem to be irritable all the time.

Martin had taken Janet to a physiatrist for evaluation and the physiatrist said he could help her. After several months Janet was showing progress and beginning slowly to be in remission. Janet still had the sleeping problem, aches and pain but she was complaining much less. One of Martin's friends suggested that she try some herbal tea with marijuana in it before she goes to sleep at night. Martin didn't like the idea of giving his wife marijuana with tea but he loves his wife and would do anything in his power to help her with her illness. So through a friend, of a friend, of a friend, Martin brought some marijuana and talked his wife into drinking green tea mixed with marijuana before her bed time. The first night after Janet had taken the herbal night cap, she slept through the night straight through to the morning without a problem. She didn't like the idea of taking marijuana at all but she was willing to try almost anything at this point. The second night she did the same thing and the next morning with the same results. It had worked for her. She was able to begin to sleep straight through the night without disturbance.

The marijuana had inhibited her dream pattern and allowed her to get a good night's sleep. After three weeks Janet was improving and began to drink hot green tea with marijuana in it in the afternoon time as well as before bed time. Her attitude was more positive and she seemed to have more energy during the course of the day. Being that Janet was well rested after several uninterrupted nights of full sleep she felt better. She lost the aches and pain and complained much less if not at all. She also began to eat more food which increases her body weight back to normal for her height. The marijuana also increases appetite. Janet began to understand the benefits of herbal medicines and began to read books on all types of medicinal herbs. As for Martin he noticed the difference in Janet within those three weeks for the better in his opinion. For Martin, these times also had become stressful for himself so Janet's improvement was a relief for him. He thought to himself that now finally he and Janet could get back to some type of normalcy. Martin was happy with the results. He was getting his wife back as she was before the illness struck her. He didn't like having to buy marijuana illegally for his wife but he would do what he would have to do to help his wife. He wished that their State had legalization of medical marijuana for medical use. Janet would continue to see the physiatrist but much less frequently, which was beneficial. Janet became more active with her daily activities as well as spending more time with Martin going to different affairs like sports events, friends get together, and others. Janet would take other herbs to help her body like horseradish, St. John's wort, mustard, allspice, kava, marijuana, devils claw, winter green, and Asian Ginseng.

Testimonials - ADHD, OCD and Personality Disorders

Ruth R. suffers from ADHD

Ruth R. is a 25 year old woman who attends college. She lives with her adoptive parents and younger adoptive brother and sister. She was adopted when she was 4 months old after child protective services removed her from her home due to physical abuse and neglect. Very little is known about the medical, psychological, and social back ground of Ruth's biological parents. Ruth R. experiences anxiety, depression and acting out behaviors. She is very disorganized, forgetful and distracted. Her parents also describe her as 'hyper'. She can't sit still and is always talking and moving around. Signs of depression, she has negative changes in mood that are powerful and pervasive. She experiences strong and frequent feelings of dejection, worthlessness, gloom about the past, hopelessness about the future and often apprehension. A complete psychological evaluation failed to confirm true attentional and consistent with an ADHD diagnosis. Psychological testing revealed below average abilities and poor feelings of anger and sadness that contributed to Ruth's poor judgment, vulnerability to peer pressure, and impulsive acting out. The psychologist conducting the evaluation suggested that Ruth would benefit from tutorial assistance at school, group therapy to assist her in contending with painful emotions related to her early history and family therapy.

Ruth meets a man in group therapy that she is very interested in. They started dating and she gets to know him better. His name is John S., he has lived in a residential care facility for the past seven years he is now 30 years old. He has had several hospitalizations in the five years prior to meeting Ruth. John takes antipsychotic medication which seems to completely control the hallucinations he experienced in the past. He now has been found to suffer from depression, OCD, and chronic back pain. John remains unable to function independently. He has been enrolled in several rehabilitative programs before he met Ruth, including sheltered workshops, but was unable to follow through with their recommendations. John also attempted to complete an associate's degree but dropped out during his first semester. Poor attendance and difficulty attending to tasks were the primary reasons for his failure. John also has great difficulty in social situations. He tends to be passive, avoiding conversation and relationships even though he says he is very lonely. john also uses herbs, herbal medicine and is a believer in holistic medicine,. He uses medical marijuana for his depression, OCD and chronic back pain which occurred after driving on a long road trip and helping to move a sofa.

John went to his physician who prescribed pain relief medications and gave him a hand out of stretches and exercises. Now, one year later thanks to the herbs and medical marijuana John is not pain free but he manages his pain without the side effects of prescription medication and pain management. As Ruth gets to know John better the closer they become, they see each other every weekend and at group therapy. Now John is no longer lonely and has developed a relationship with Ruth. Over dinner one evening John told Ruth to try some medical marijuana to help her anxiety and depression. Ruth trusted John and she knew he was into herbs and herbal medicine. She saw how it helped his condition, she tried some in tea and smoked it. She felt relief right away, and after a while she could see and feel the difference. Ruth is not as anxious or depressed as she used to be. She knew it was the medical marijuana, it also helped her hyperactivity without the side effects of her prescribed medications. Ruth improved so much she applied for a deli position at a local supermarket, and to her surprise, she was hired. Ruth's case manager is an occupational therapist who regularly checks on her wellbeing on her job and provides employment supports for Ruth when she needs them. Job related issues come up on a regular basis, but consistent support in her employment has helped Ruth manage her symptoms, develop her problem solving skills, and fully utilize all the resources she has available to her.

Lois G. suffers with OCD

This story is from Lois G. that suffers with Obsessive Compulsive Disorder; My name is Lois G., I am an 30 year old female, married with OCD. When I was a teenager, I had all kinds of fear. I didn't want to go outside, I couldn't fall asleep at night because b I was afraid I was going to die. I even stopped eating at one point, because I thought that the food would stick in my throat and I would choke. I saw a psychiatrist who told my parents that I was simply afraid to grow up. My parents didn't have any idea about what was going on with me. We lived on an air force base, and they took me to lots of doctors who didn't have a clue about what might be causing my strange behavior. I remember one doctor who asked me why I wouldn't eat. I told him if I eat, I would choke and die. He only wanted to know about my family relationships and whether or not I got along with my mother and father. I didn't have a problem with my parents, we were a very loving family. I lost so much weight that I was hospitalized. I was given a lot of medical tests, which proved that there was nothing blocking my throat. My would tell me over and over again that there was no reason for me to be afraid of choking. They began treating me for anorexia nervosa, which is not what I had at all. It was a very frustrating time for me. Things were very tough in our family because no one understood me. During my teenage years. I saw social workers, therapists, psychiatrists, and psychologists. They all tried to figure out what was going on with me, but no one came up with an answer. My parents were told to wait it out, that it was just something I would have to outgrow. Despite all the help my parents were trying to get for me, nothing was actually working.

I had so many fears that, at one point, I couldn't be around other people. I didn't even want to go to school. My parents threaded to send me away to boarding school, which was a hard idea to me. Instead I attended a local program for kids who needed a different atmosphere from the regular high school, and it seemed just perfect. I fit in there very well.

Within a year, I was able to return to my high school and graduate. When I went to college, my symptoms got worse again. I had new fears. I could manage on the outside, but back in my apartment, I would fall apart and worry about everything. I saw a social worker who thought that I was afraid of graduating and having to enter the real world. He told me that I should just get married and have ten kids, so that I wouldn't have time to worry. I just kept most of my worries to myself because they were very scary. I thought I was either going to go crazy or that people would think I was crazy if I told them what was v in my mind.

I met my husband Les when I was in college. I purposely didn't tell him about symptoms. I hid them from him. I told him about my fear of driving and that I needed to check and recheck that I hadn't run over someone with my car. I was afraid Les would say I was crazy. A few years later I finally found out what was wrong with me.

One day at work I was reading a Times magazine article about obsessive-compulsive disorder. I remember leaving the office with the magazine, thinking, "this is it! I'm not crazy, I have OCD. I wished I had looked for another therapist right then and showed her the article, but it would be another five years before that happened.

Les and I had gotten married and we had three children. I had a very bad bout of OCD a year after our second child was born. At times, no one besides Les knew that I had this illness. Things got so bad that I finally called my mother and pleaded with her to help me take care of the kids. I had hit rock- bottom. I tearfully told Les that I thought I might need to tell someone the truth about what I was struggling with and that maybe I should start taking medication. I met with another therapist, and this time, I cried my heart out to her. She said "you're not crazy". She was the first mental health professional in all these years who gave me a diagnosis. This was the first time I felt safe enough to actually talk about my obsessions and compulsions and rituals with a therapist.

My ultimate fear was that I would lose my children. My kids are my life. After I was diagnosed, Les kept urging me to tell my family about my OCD. I didn't want anyone to know about my illness because I still felt that in some way I wasn't made of the right stuff. I was afraid that people even my family members, would relate to me differently if they knew about my OCD. When I finally did tell my mom and sisters, all they wanted to know was how they could help me. My diagnosis explained so much about my strange behavior back when I was a teenager. It took me much longer before I told Les family that I had OCD. I have the kind of OCD where I do a lot of checking. For instance, when I leave the house in the morning, I have to follow a certain pattern. I have to check the stove, the coffee pot, the toaster, and the oven. Even if I know that I haven't used the stove. I still have to make sure that it's turned off. I check the appliances three or four times. When I was at my worst a few years ago, I would have checked maybe five, six, or seven times, left the house and locked the door, gone down the steps, and then unlocked door, gone back into the kitchen, and made sure yet again that everything was unplugged. Even then in my n mind I would doubt whether I had really checked everything or not.

After I was diagnosed, I read about OCD, but for a long time, I never met or talked to anybody else who had it. I decided to join a support group for people who have this illness. One day in group therapy, one woman from the group asked to speak to me alone. She told me about medical marijuana I was very surprised but I kept listening, she explained how antidepressants and medical marijuana helped her so much with her OCD. So I decided to try it. I told my husband he was against it at first but after I kept on him about it, he agreed I should try it. What a difference! Almost immediately I felt relaxed and in control, my OCD was under control for the first time in years. I could do things that I hadn't been able to do for years without so much as a worry. The more I understand about OCD and other mental illnesses, the more compassion I feel for others who suffer from these disorders. I have compassion for the person living on the street who have lost their support system and is so isolated that either they don't want help or people just aren't coming to help them. Sometimes I think about how different my life would have been if I didn't have OCD. But despite all the problems it has cause, I've pretty much decided that having OCD is not the worst thing that can happen to you. Over the years I began to see my illness in a different way. I've gotten to the point where I can talk publicly about having OCD. I work as an advocate for the national alliance for the mentally ill. People do look at you differently when you have a mental illness or any other "abnormal" condition. Fortunately, I'm not one to worry about what other people think about my family or about me.

Jake W. has a HYPERACTIVE PERSONALITY

There is a young man named Jake W. that has hyperactive personality and has a anger management problem. He takes all the worlds untruths as a personal betrayal which makes him angry. He gets disgusted with all the injustice in the country and he world. He sees all the wrongs that are being excepted and none of the rights be pronounced. He would let some things upset him were the average person would ignore. Jake is the type of person that people would say, he has a head full of bad wiring. Jake would buy marijuana and use it as a anger management medication that kept him calm and relax and not taking a personal interest in the world's problems. Jake was able to concentrate his thinking on things that are more important to his life as well as make judgment calls on important decisions without anger being a factor. He seemed to have more of a positive personality after taking marijuana as a medication. Not saying that marijuana solved all his problems but it helped him deal with them better. It was hard for Jake to maintain a steady relationship with a woman because of his anger. He had several relationships but none of them lasted for any length of time. He would not be able to control his anger and become verbally abusive to whatever woman he was with at the time. Jake could be helped with psychiatric canceling and should get some. Jake would have to deal with his own personal problems before he could really have a steady relationship with a woman. Jake would have to learn about himself to correct his own faults no matter how many there are and how long it takes.

Testimonials - Paranoid Schizoaffective and Schizophrenia
Marie G. suffers from PARANOID SCHIZOAFFECTIVE DISORDER

Marie G. is a 35 year old female diagnosed with paranoid schizoaffective disorder, who lives with her husband James, and their 2- year old son Timmy. Marie's mother received a telephone call one morning from James who told her that Marie was up all night changing clothes and now she's mad at him and talking weird.

James and Maries mother got together to get her the help she needed. They got her a case manager who addressed her medication and living skills training and weekly home visits. The case manager, who was familiar with Marie's pattern of relapse and an extra staff person is helpful for support in a crisis situation. At the home the case manager and Marie's husband found Marie dressed bizarrely with short tight clothing, with very heavy make-up and black nail polish. She was agitated and pacing, her speech was rapid and was coupled with hostile stares and verbally a bused the case manager saying things like "you're all made of wax and you're going to die in the nuclear meltdown". Shouting and screaming obscenities. She couldn't talk to her case manager as she continued to pace, stopping occasionally to stare at the case manager and social worker making bizarre accusations.

A few weeks later Marie started with the help of her social worker a learning styles approach. She was then more able to decide which groups and treatment approaches would most likely to interest her and which would most likely be difficult. A few weeks later Marie drove to the Mall she began to feel ill, she drove back home gasping for air running from across the yard, James found her bent over gasping for breath. Marie's heart was racing and she felt dizzy. James helped her to the house and called the doctor. Marie was feeling better by the time they arrived at the office, the doctor ran a number of tests over the next several weeks. During that time, Marie continued to have occasional episodes. The tests came back negative for a physical cause for Marie's symptoms.

As time passed, Marie became increasingly fearful of going anywhere alone. What if she had one of the episodes and no one was around to help her? Until now, she had recovered within a few minutes, but what if help wasn't available, she was alone, and she didn't recover so quickly. She could die alone with no one to help her. Marie also feared the humiliation of having an episode in public. It was terribly embarrassing. She'd feel the stares of people who wondered what was wrong, what they can do to help. Marie was sure many thought she was just trying to draw attention to herself. She confided in two close friends besides James and made them promise to stay with her as much as possible. James and Marie had married in their early 20s. Marie had been a flight attendant but quit when she married. James wanted his wife home with him every evening. Marie also couldn't bear the separations at that time and happily shifted to a job at the local hospital. Within a year, Marie began to miss the freedom, excitement, and respect that she had enjoyed with her last job. She felt constantly constricted.

Every time she suggested a job change, James started criticizing her. He would say that she didn't know how to create a good home or appreciate all that they did have. Eventually she had Timmy and quit work to be a full-time home maker. With the arrival of Timmy, James quickly became unable to share any of his feelings or thoughts with Marie. He came home, played with Timmy and watched TV. The only time he touched Marie was in bed for sexual intercourse. Marie could not stand his anger. Her anger seethed all day and night, and once a week, usually on the weekend, she confronted him. He usually listened for a minute and then walked out of the room. Then he ignored her for the rest of the night or became totally absorbed in a book or a game with Timmy. At times, Marie felt he did little things to retaliate for her out bursts, such as refusing to get out a video that she was looking forward to seeing or making fun of her friends.

The other trigger that really got to Marie was that James did not help with any of the house work. He felt that because he was the sole breadwinner, her job was to cook, clean, pay the bills, do, the repairs, and organize Timmy's actives. If they were going to have people over for the evening, James would be sure to come home from work or his weekend exercise routine just when the guests arrived. When Marie tried to get James involved, he simple stated that he was not going to do it and she should just get used to that fact. After one child and years of Marriage, Marie was angry nearly all of the time. Eventually, she started a children's birthday party business and increasing contact with families with young children convinced her she needed to be in therapy. The other woman she met seemed so care free and happy with their husbands and their lives. She realized for the first time, that she had been getting less than she felt she deserved from her marriage. Marie was in therapy only a month when James decided to come and see what she was wasting all the money on. James showed a complete denial of any anger or distancing. He thought if Marie could only stop taking life so seriously, they would get along fine. He admitted that he didn't want to do any house work and felt justified that the traditional division of labor was fair in their case. Several weeks later Marie's mother was at the salon getting her hair done. Her mother started talking about her daughter and what she was going through. Her hair stylist suggested marijuana because it helped her with her depression. She arranged to pick up some medical marijuana from her stylist. Marie's mother got her to try it, and it made all the difference. Marie became more assertive and confident. She began to explain, why she was asking for James help with house work. Her major point was that house work was an expression of her commitment to the marriage and family. She refused to accept it as her job. Slowly and without ever admitting he was changing James started asking her what he could do for her around the house so that she could stop seeing the shrink. Now Marie felt James was on her side. She knew he was becoming aware of what she was feeling, and this made all the difference in the world to her. Six months after taking the medical marijuana James and Marie started couples therapy, their marriage strengthened. James started balancing the attention he gave Timmy with the attention he gave his wife. Even though they still have minor disagreements, they were always resolved before the night was over.

Jeff S. suffers from PARANOID SCHIZOPHRENIA

My name is Jeff S. I was diagnosed with paranoid schizophrenia when I was only twenty two years old. For the next ten years I was in and out of various mental hospitals. I was told many times that I was insane, and I was given little hope that I could ever lead a dignified or reasonably normal life. Today I work for a psychiatric hospital in Denver. My first breakdown occurred when I was an officer in the Navy, responsible for the security of powerful weapons. It was a stressful job, and I felt under pressure. After nine months on assignment, I began to believe that enemies of our country had hypnotized certain officers and that they were planning to use their power to threaten our national security. So I shared this information with the psychiatrist at the hospital on the base. After listening to me, he told me I would be staying in the hospital. I was led into a padded room, the door was locked and I was left all alone. I believed the psychiatrist was sure that I would be shot and killed. I spent the next five months in a locked psychiatric unit, where I was given powerful tranquilizers. I was in anguish from the side effects. I resisted them. Eventually I gradually improved. When I left the hospital, I was able to look briefly at my medical record. I was surprised and upset to see v many negative comments about my family. Upon my release from the hospital I was discharged from the Navy. While I was hospitalized several of my fellow patents were kind enough to sign letters of recommendation for me so I could apply for admission to a graduate school in international business. I was accepted. I didn't tell anyone there what had happened to me. No one knew anything about my psychiatric history. I graduated with a business degree and received several job offers. I accepted one with a Fortune 500 company and was planning to live my life " happily ever after". It didn't turn out that way. I had another breakdown after three months on the job and wound up back in a psychiatric ward of a county hospital. When I was released a few weeks later, I was still delusional. Even though I was able to return to work, it was obvious to the management of the company that I was quite sick. One day at work. I found myself barking and growling as though I was an animal. Eventually one of my relatives flew from his house in Texas to help me. I went to Texas with him, where I was returned into a hospital. When I was discharged I went to stay with my parents in Florida. I spent most of my time there in bed because when I was awake, my life was too painful for me to face.

I began to feel a little better after a few months, so I stopped taking my medication. I decided to leave my parents home and went to Ohio to live. I found a job as a real estate salesman, but after working for several months, I had made no sales and earned no money. I had yet another breakdown. I became delusional and was behaving bizarrely for about three weeks. I was admitted to the local state hospital and committed as an "insane person." I was soon transferred to a VA hospital, where I stayed for two months, while I was there a young intern told me I could have gone far in life if it weren't for my mental condition, which was right. This made me want to succeed in life.

When I was discharged this time, I was able to find a job working in a nearby maximum sec. unity psychiatric hospital. At that time I passed a civil service examination that qualified me for the position. I was well enough to stay out of the hospital for three years. Then I returned to graduate school, this time course work for both my masters and my PHD. I continued to be psychologically fragile and had two more hospitalizations while I was in graduate school. The last one was in 1974. Soon after I met my wife Karen when I was in graduate school. I liked her a lot, I assumed she was married because she was wearing a ring. But one day Karen told me that the ring signified that she was a Franciscan Nun. I was very much taken aback by this news, but probably no more surprised than Karen was when I told her a few weeks later that I had schizophrenia. Less than a year later, the beautiful lady who had entered a convent fifteen years earlier and the man who had repeatedly been put away in mental hospitals were married. I still have to take antipsychotic medication, but I now take medical marijuana and that makes all the difference. I was first introduced to marijuana when I was in the service. Without medical marijuana I would be back on a locked ward. So I take it daily. It helps me stay calm, relaxed and not anxious. Knowing that there is a strong genetic component to mental illness, I was not totally surprised. When our daughter Beth, began having emotional difficulties and went on medication. Beth has severe depression. When Jeff and I took our daughter to see her pediatrician for help he told us ' give her warm milk and keep her on a specific schedule. He thought her insomnia was causing all of her problems. Her sleep patterns never varied, but it did not make any difference. By this time Beth was threatening suicide almost daily. We took her to a therapist, who told us she needs medication and there was an instant change in her for the better.

All four of our children have varying degrees of depression and they have all been on antidepressants. Our daughter Beth, has had the toughest time of it she was only eleven. When she was diagnosed. She always had troubling symptoms. When she was diagnosed, she always had troubling symptoms. Mental illness is like a black hole, sometimes I feel like I'm being sucked in and can't get out. Fortunately not everybody in our family has episodes simultaneously. Our friends and family members are pretty compassionate and understanding. I worried that people would think that I was weird because I had a mental illness. I would see movies or television shows that portrayed people with mental illnesses killers or as so strange that no one could believe they were really human. I don't want people to think of me that way. I doesn't like having schizophrenia or depression, it made me tired and cranky, and I can't be the person I want to be. I wish nothing bad ever happened to me or my family members, but everyone has their cross to bear. I'm just lucky that my family is able to cope with mental illness as well as they do. When I applied to college, I didn't see a reason to hide my mental illness. I had of my depression, which I got with no contest. I had a reputation on campus for being very open about my mental illness. I've never encountered any sort of negative reaction at all. I had a reputation on campus for being very open about my mental illness. I've never encountered any sort of negative reaction at all. I'm fine as long as I'm on my meds and medical marijuana which is the right combination for me. I sleep better, and things turned around immediately, my life got better. Now I'm a speaker and advocate in the schools with educational videos about mental illness.

George E. suffers from SCHIZOPHRENIA

My name is George E. 26 years of age. I have a twin brother, we both have Schizophrenia and this is our story. I live in my own apartment near by my twin Jerry. Jerry is married and has a child. I first realized that I might be sick when I was a teenager. I was confused, I couldn't think straight. There was something wrong with my head. I started to talk about these religious with my head. I started to talk about these religious delusions I was having.

Within weeks I was tested by a psychologist, who diagnosed me as having latent schizophrenia. I was admitted into a psychiatric hospital almost immediately. I came home early one night from playing in a varsity football game. I was telling my twin brother that when I was on the field, I had this delusion that I didn't have any clothes on. I tried to get hurt so that I could get off the field because I thought everybody was staring at me. George didn't want to tell anyone what was happening to him. Jerry followed George into the hospital. We were depressed and sick, but we both got good care. Jerry and I both got a pass from our psychiatrist to leave the hospital to go to their senior prom. My twin and I were hospitalized for six months. When we were released and returned home we didn't know how to manage. We were like little birds that wanted to grow up and jump out of the nest.

George worked as a security guard for a while. Then I joined the Navy. A Navy hospital in Chicago admitted me to their psychiatric unit. I had cracked up just two days after my enlistment. After they stabilized me, the Navy sent me home with a honorable discharge. People have to get educated and learn about how to survive. Now I give back what I've learned. I get a big thrill out of helping other people. My twin and I go on panels to educate professionals about how families cope with mental illness. My twin and I didn't want to take our medications at first. We would be released from the hospital and then forget to take our meds and end up right back in the hospital. It would be turmoil all over again trying to get stabilized. There were always setbacks for us. These days I get together with my twin once in a while. If I have a barbecue, I'll ask him over we've gone camping and to the movies. If I need to move furniture or something like that, I'll ask him to help me. I know I can always count on him. We're still close even though we do our own thing. I never get disappointed with him if he can't handle something, because I know it's his mental illness,. People need to know what having Schizophrenia is really like, just the facts. The real version, not the Hollywood one. With Schizophrenia, when you're not on your medication, you have delusions, you have paranoia, your moods go up and down, you hear voice. You're pretty much out there. You just don't know what's going on. When you're mentally ill, you're living in a science fiction world that's come true.

It was not easy was reluctant at first, but I decided to try it. Along with our regular medication, the herbal medication for me to take my meds but it is vitally important for me to do so. At first I refused because I didn't think I was sick. I take my meds regularly not and

I don't need reminders any more. My twin convinced me to see Chinese herbal doctors and medical marijuana. I was reluctant at first, but I decided to try it. Along with our regular medication.

The herbal medicines help us remain calm and stable. My twin and I accepted these medicines because they worked for us. OF all the things I do to help my twin brother, none of them compare with the support of family and close friends. When I learned that my twin and I would never be cured my family never questioned their decision to care for us. They give us the moral support to go on. We were also fortunate to find a friendly church whose members care for us. Their caring was an open demonstration of acceptance and brotherly love. They helped my brother and I rebuild our faith and trust in other people. It touched both of us. My twin and I love to go hiking, climb mountains and go camping with groups because that improves our health. The beautiful scenery helps me open my heart. I have a good time talking with friends, and this helps me get away from loneliness. Sometimes I work as a volunteer to build and maintain trails with my brother. I feel that I'm very useful and that all the activity is helpful for my illness. When I first got sick I was about sixteen and a half. I was in high school. I had no idea what was happening to me and even now, there's a lot I don't remember. For years, I was always in and out of the hospital every few months because I would stop taking my meds. I'm thirty-seven now and thanks to medical marijuana and herbal medicine I haven't been in the hospital for three years. I've been married and divorced twice. I have a twelve year-old son who lives with his mom. My twin brother and I are really close. Even though Jerry is married now and has a two-month-old daughter, we've stuck together. I've become an advocate for the mentally ill. When I first started working at the clinic. My doctor asked me if I had ever made a speech. I said no, and he said "we'll have you speaking all over the place." And I have! I average eight appearances a year at conferences and at law enforcement agencies. I explained that even an over achiever like me can become mentally ill. I tell the audiences that I was the student body president in high school and an excellent student all though college. Mental illness does not affect just one type of person. After I spoke to one police department, they came

191

up with the idea of making cards like drivers licenses that would identify a person as mentally ill. The purpose of these I D cards is to save people's lives. Folks who have mental illness are often jailed and then kill themselves there. The police don't usually realize that a prisoner is sick until after the fact. If the police were informed, these folks could be sent to a special place where they could receive treatment. I hope one day there would be a cure for mental illness. It's just a matter of time and research. Maybe someday the whole mental health system will be out of business. I like to give people hope that if I can get well, so can they. I'm now able to work part-time at the clinic where I used to be a mental health consumer. I'm not working full- time yet, but I will sometimes soon I'm just not ready for that yet. Many people won't tell anyone that someone in their family has a mental illness. They keep it to themselves and hibernate in a closet. I tell people like that to open up and let the world know. Treat the mentally as normally as anybody else. Don't treat them differently. I never thought about mental illness before I got sick. It never even crossed my mind. Because our family hadn't ever experienced it. Everything was new to us. After I was diagnosed, I started reading books and watching television shows about mental illness.

It's sad that the only way people will reach out and do anything about mental illness is when it hits someone in their own family. Before I learned about mental illness I was ignorant of the facts. I didn't even know what mental illness was. I thought that all people who were mentally ill had gone through bad experiences, which made them go over the edge. What really gets me upset is when researchers find a medication that works well, but there aren't enough people who need it. Then the drug companies don't want to spend the money making it because they can't make a big enough profit. This is called an "orphan medication". I call it corporate greed.

Atopic Dermatitis

ATOPIC DERMATITIS

Atopic Dermatitis is a skin inflammation that causes intense itching and discomfort. It is a chronic, inherited skin disorder in which the immune system produces a hypersensitivity reaction to environmental allergens. This inherited disorder reoccurs throughout the patient's life. Scratching the skin causes vasoconstriction and intensifies pruritus, resulting in erythematous and lesions. A patient that has a history of atopy, such as allergic rhinitis asthma, or urticaria. Some family members may have a similar history. To treat this chronic disorder includes skin care, environmental control of allergens and drug therapy. Some patients are taking medical marijuana for the discomfort and as a relaxer to relieve stress.

Testimonials - Dermatitis

Edward T. suffers from DERMATITIS

Edward T. suffers from Dermatitis (Inflammation of the skin and various skin lesions) all of his life. He is 22 years old living with his parents and younger sister and works at a department store full time. Edward's particular type of Dermatitis is Herpetiformis. He's had this skin disorder all of his life. Throw out the years he has learned how to take care of his skin disorder with antiseptic lotions, discomfort medications. When Edward was younger at the age of 8 he had a traumatic experience playing with other children the same age. We all know that some children can be cruel to each other for whatever reason. This particular day a few of the children started to pick on and tease Edward about his skin rash and constant scratching. Edward's skin disorder would make him scratch his skin due to itching and the burning feeling. That particular day the children's teasing was indelibly imprinted in Edward's mind. This hurt Edward's feelings and he would never forget it. From then on he would always be conscious of his skin appearance and how it looked to other people.

Edward soon realized that he shouldn't always worry about what other people think of his skin disorder. He learned that other people would accept him for the good person that he was, and those people that didn't see him for the good person that he was and only saw his rash didn't really know him. Edward found it hard to meet young ladies because of his rash so he relied on his sparkling personality and wit to meet young ladies. Edward seems to know everyone in his school and was popular with his class mates.

As a teenager he would try to act and look likes the other teenagers that he would hang out with. When his group of teenagers were out of school at the end of the day, they would either play video games, or party at each other's house when only the parents of the house they chose was not home. Each of their houses has a play room or den that had a big TV and video game set, or pool table, or card table or something else. Edward and his friends would do whatever event they wanted to do at these parties including drinking alcohol and all types of drugs. These teenagers are what's called street savvy and have experimented with all the illegal drugs on the market at one time or another. These teenagers have chosen marijuana as the only drug they would take at these parties, calling them pot parties. These teenagers all are having passing grades in school and stay out of trouble. These teenagers are basically the normal good teenagers and all their parents know this. The parents of these teenagers know that their children are hanging out together at each other's houses and they don't mind that. The parents feel that it is better for their children to hang out at each other's house rather than hanging out at clubs, bars, or on the streets. The teenager's parents communicate with each other and know what their teenagers are doing and where they are.

The parents are aware that their teenagers are smoking marijuana at these get together and don't like it but in their minds they where rather have their teenagers smoking marijuana than possibly smoking crack or taking the other types of illegal street drugs out there. The parents considered marijuana less of a evil than the other habit forming street drugs that are 100 times more dangerous. The parents knew that marijuana was not habit forming and consider it as just going through a teenage faze. As for Edward, marijuana has much more benefits than just a party drug. For him marijuana helped him to deal with his lifelong Dermatitis disorder. For Edward marijuana had become medical marijuana because it has helped him medically, and has become a part of his treatment for his Dermatitis disorder. Edward was less conscious of his daily discomfort of itching and burning sensation when taking medical marijuana. Edward would add medical marijuana to the daily medication and skin lotions he would take to treat his Dermatitis disorder even up to now. These are other herbal medications that treat this disorder. Gota Kola, cleavers, aloe vera, papaya, ivy, and allspice.

<u>Sleep Disorders</u>

Testimonials - Sleep Disorders

Dylan L. suffers from INSOMNIA

Dylan L. suffers from Insomnia, (can't sleep) which is affecting his job performance. Dylan is a Lawyer involved in corporate law and works for several different corporate firms. It is a stressful and pressure induced profession for some. Dylan deals with corporate cases involving hundreds of millions of dollars. So he constantly works late into the night and gets up early to prepare for court. When Dylan would go to his bed, he didn't go to sleep right away. His mind was still working overtime before he fell asleep for the night. Some nights he can't go to sleep at all and other nights he gets 3 to 5 hours of sleep. Other nights he would close his eyes for what seem like 5 minutes and he open his eyes and it was time to get up. Dylan could be considered a workaholic or just dedicated to his work. Dylan couldn't afford to make erase in the court room due to lack of sleep. So he tried taking sleeping pills but that seem to make him slow and groggy in the mornings, so that didn't work and he stopped taking them. One day Dylan's girl friend suggested that he try some herbal tea mixed with marijuana to help him go to sleep at night. The next day Dylan's girl friend brought him some herbal tea mixed with marijuana.

She told Dylan to make the hot herbal tea mix, and drink it a half hour before going to bed. She also said, of course you have to go to bed at a decent time to bet enough sleep hours for his body, in other words get bed early. So Dylan did what she said and it worked.

195

He got full night's sleep and felt good with no after effect. From then on Dylan would take the herbal tea and marijuana mix to aid his insomnia and help him in his normal life. There were times when Dylan did not have insomnia during this short period. He would start to take less herbal tea mix every week until he was taking it three times a week. Dylan began to have more energy during the course of a normal day. He was able to concentrate better and make less mistakes and better decisions during the course of a day. Dylan's life was improving on a daily bases and he didn't look back. That was five years ago and now Dylan is happily married to his then girl friend and still takes the herbal tea and marijuana mix. Other herbs taken are, Humulus- lupulus, Hypericum perforatum, Lavandula angustifolia, Melissa officinalis,.

Barbara W. suffers from MULTIPLE ILLNESSES

Barbara W. is a 55 year old that suffered from multiple illnesses. She just buried her son one year ago that was killed in the war. But for Barbara it was like yesterday. A person can never get over the hurt of having to bury their own child, before their own demise. For Barbara a large part of herself had died to. She struggle to keep her sanity after being notified of her son's death. Barbara is still in the morning stage of the loss of her son and she may never ever get over it. Barbara has post-traumatic stress disorder. The traumatic incident of her son being killed in the war haunts her. Of cause the grief was over whelming for her. She has many sleepless nights due to nightmares. These nightmares consisted of different cinereous of Barbara witnesses her son's death in the war. She said each nightmare was different but similar and always ended up with the same results, her son's death. During the day many things remind her of her son, whether it be places, things or even dates. She would take marijuana before bed time to stop the nightmares and get a better night's sleep . She did not want her son to go to war but there was nothing she could do to stop him. This was something he felt he had to do so he did.

James C. is a PARAPLEGIC

James C. is a 32 year old Paraplegic that lost his legs in the war four years ago. James had join the military seven years ago with the energy and spirit to be a good soldier and what's called an all American boy that loves his country and would give up his life to defend it. James was the type of soldier that always completed whatever task set before him. One day he and his men were escorting a convoy of trucks with supplies from one town to another town in the mid east when the convoy was attacked with R-P-G fire and road side bombs. In that attack on the convoy most of James's fellow soldiers were killed and he lost his legs that day and still lived. Since the time he lost his legs he has found it difficult to make the adjustment of being a paraplegic and continuing with life. James had felt that he should have died with his men that day but that wasn't to be, he was to live. James has a lot of mental such as nightmares of war that he has often and frequently of horrifying situations which is partly due to his subconscious or feelings of guilt.

James is married with two children, and eight year old boy named Jimmy and a nine year old daughter named Lisa. Both children are very proud of their father and his sacrifice for them and the country. James wife's name is Lesley who was James salvation in this four year time period after losing his legs. Once James came back from overseas to the United States. Lesley was right there to help and take care of her man. James is very lucky to have such a loving family that love him so much so as to except his misfortune. James is happy to be home and yet he has feelings of fear of his families future and how he could continue to support them. James was receiving military benefits for himself and his family and yet he still has fears. James is using a wheelchair to get a round and with a lot of aid from his family . These days James has bouts with depression that come and go. He tries to hide his moments of depression from his family but his wife Lesley can always tell. James would be depressed when he could not do the thing he use to do when he had his legs. Like playing with his children, going up stairs, or even a little walk down the street. The things we all take for granted when we have legs to walk with. James would take marijuana to help him sleep and with bouts depression which helped him maintain himself. James was on the list to receive a pair of new state of the art bionic legs from a governmental organization program. These bionic legs work by attaching sensors to implants in his legs to transmit and receive information to the legs from the leg muscle. This technology is also augmented with a micro computer system. This is new technology will enable James to walk again or even possibly run again. James was looking forward to receiving the new bionic legs and being able to stand up on two feet and walk once again. He would have to wait a little longer when he is next on the list.

James would investigate and get information about the bionic legs system and how they work with his limbs. He would get this information from his doctor. This gave James hope for the future and something good to look forward to. He would still take marijuana to help with his nightmares. When James turn came he was prepared on the procedure that entailed with the insertions of the sensors and there functions in regards to the legs system. The procedure would take over a half dozen sessions and appointments to fine tune his legs system to function correctly. At first James's family were expecting him to just get up and walk, hop, skip and jump the same day but James would have to learn how to balance while standing up. And then he would have to learn how to walk, one step at a time. James would have to start over at the beginning and practice every day. It took a few days of learning how to stand with his new legs and a few weeks for him to learn how to walk again. Once he was confident with his walking abilities he would venture out into the world on his own without the assistance of a wheelchair or assistance from others. He could now do some of the things he use to do in the past like playing with his children or shopping with his wife at the local mall. Or going out for dinner and a movie show or sports event. James would have to go constantly back and forth to the doctors for fine adjustments to the bionic system incorporated with his body. At first when James started learning how to walk again he looked very mechanical in his movement and motion. Like a robot, stiff and uncoordinated. So it took some fine tuning by the doctors and a lot of practice by James so he could walk fluently. The children would tease James by calling him bionic daddy. James would get a kick out of that and laugh about it. The children felt even more proud of their farther and admired his bravery being a test subject for bionics. James would still take marijuana to relax and to be able to sleep through the night. As time moves on James would not need the marijuana as a sleep aid anymore and have no habit forming effects of withdrawal like some other sleep AIDS. James got his life back and was grateful to everyone that had helped him through the whole ordeal during the years after losing his legs in the war.

Helen H. is a PARAPLEGIC

Helen H. is a 29 year old paraplegic that lost the use of her legs due to a car accident in which her husband was killed three years prior. Losing her husband and becoming a paraplegic has changed her life in major was. It's been three years since the accident and Helen has made great strides in accepting her losses but she still has a long way to go. Her mental condition was very depressed and at times suicidal. Helen's family and friends always made sure to include Helen in all events and affairs so she would not feel alone and excluded. Helen received a large settlement in he death of her husband and the loss of the use of her legs. She has a health attendant as well and occasional nurse to help out and take care of her. Helen did not like the depression medication that was prescribed for her by a doctor or certain pain medicine she was taking. She had read that medical marijuana could help her with some discomfort so she so she asked her brother to get her some to see if marijuana could help her. Helen began to become more hopeful and optimistic about her future and began to savor life and it's special moments. It was very hard for her to overcome her tragedies but she is doing it every day. Helen said that one day, she was in the depth of depression, feeling the lowest a person could feel. Letting her feelings control her mind which is a mistake. She smoked some marijuana and she began to think differently and feel better. She would stop thinking selfishly and more grateful to still be alive. She would hold these thoughts even after the affects of the marijuana have dissipated. When Helen was comfortable with her motorized wheelchair she would go out shopping with her aid, to the clinic, or doctors office, or therapy session. Helen's attitude changed for the better she would exercise to improve so may take better care of herself. She began to became stronger and more self positive and independent. She also spent some time painting pictures and starting a career as an artist. Helen never realized that she had this hidden talent with a paint brush. Maybe now that she has more time on her hands she's able to take a good look at her options.

Testimonials - Severe Burns

Gordon L. is a BURN PATIENT

Gordon L. is a 42 year old burn patient that was in a fire seven years ago that had 40% of his body burned. He has gone through dozens of skin grafts on his face and different parts of his body. His whole life had changed after the fire. Gordon was a TV news cast speaker before the fire. He could no longer be a TV news caster after he recuperated from being a fire burn patient so he would seek other employment as a writer of the news in a small local news paper company. Gordon would have pain and discomfort for the rest of his life. He would deal with it with different pain medications including marijuana Gordon also found out that some people would treat him differently when they saw the burns scares on his face. This would hurt his feelings sometimes but he would understand why some people would stare at him or look away. As time moves on even this would pass. Life is hard enough and for some even harder for people such as Gordon. Though out the last years Gordon went through self pity, depression, and all the other problems that a person would go through in a similar situation. Gordon's family would help him during these times with his needs. He would do all the things that a person would do in his situation and adapt to it.

Testimonials - Other Wounds or Injuries

Adam T. suffers from WAR INJURIES

Adam T. is 25 years old soldier that has return from his second tour in the war in Iraq. He was massively injured when his vehicle was attacked by a sniper and he was shot in the face. He had major facial injuries and needed facial reconstruction. Before Adam was injured he was engaged to be married and a handsome man. He had never gave a thought about his appearance, but now he does. His fiancée had left him and he was recuperating in a military hospital State side. While in this hospital he had 8 surgeries on his face only and he still feels he has to cover his face with a mask, so as not to offend anybody. After being in the military hospital for almost 2years and 15 facial surgeries he was due to be released in a few weeks. He was to go to stay with his parents at their home and they would see to his needs. Adam was afraid of leaving the sanctuary of the hospital and going out into the world once again. Adam's personality had change from being outgoing and active to the opposite. He had become withdrawn and depressed. When the time came for Adam to leave the hospital he had mustered up enough courage to leave and go home with his parents. He was still wearing the mask to cover his face as a form of security for him. He was given numerous medication and was scheduled for hospital checkups once a month. Adam's mental condition was somewhat stable considering his situation. The facial reconstruction was done with state of the art equipment and his face did not look to disfigured. But in Adam's mind he looked like the Frankenstein monster. But all of this was all in his mind. Adam's face look like a face with a lot of scares on it. It was the type of facial scares that a person get when they have been in a car accident and went through the windshield glass. Joe S. was Adam's army buddy in the hospital, after one month of Adam being home Joe contacted Adam and they got together over Joe's apartment. Adam and Joe were very close in the hospital. Joe was missing a leg in the war so they had a lot in commend. Joe is the type of person that always seems to be in a good optimistic mood all the time. Joe felt that losing his leg in the war was a small price to pay instead of his life. Adam and Joe would drink beer and talk about old times and their future. Joe being the optimistic one of the two would constantly puss Adam to do things and go places and try to meet new people to befriend. Joe would get Adam marijuana to help him relax. At first the marijuana made Adam feel more paranoid but after a short time Adam over came feeling paranoid and would relax his mind. Adam's personality began to change and get back to the way he use to be before his facial injury.

Joe and Adam would go to parties, clubs, and bars to meet woman and sometimes get lucky. One day Adam asked Joe, where do you get the marijuana from? Joe said, I have a medical marijuana card given to me by the State with my doctor's authorization to treat my depression after losing my leg. Joe said to Adam, you might be eligible to get the medical marijuana card by contacting your doctor and applying to the State. Adam was able to show just cause for acquiring a medical marijuana card. He would be able to buy medical marijuana from a State approved agency or grow it his self. For the first two months Adam brought the medical marijuana from a State agency and he decided to try to grow it at home to save money. Adam thought that it cost him over $100. For a few grams of good State agency medical marijuana ever month so he saved all the seeds he got that was in the marijuana he got each month. He brought a few books on the subject of how to grow marijuana and began to study them and learn how to grow it. He selected a location in his back yard that was out of the way and secure from others. Adam started by using a growing starter kit that he brought with all the necessary products to grow the plants. Adam knew that it would take some time for the plants to grow and mature so he still brought the State agency medical marijuana for some time. Ever time when Adam would go to buy the State agency medical marijuana he would think to himself that the State was making a lot of tax money on the sale of medical marijuana and that it was a wise thing to do to make revenue. After 5 to 6 months Adam finally had grown something. He started growing about a hundred marijuana seeds that started to come up but that soon started dying off, for one reason or another. After he had separated the male plants from the female plants and he was left with 10 female plants. Reading in one of his books told him to get rid of the male plants and keep the female plants, so he did. Adam would put his attention on the female plants to help them grow. Every week Adam would sample the plants to see how potent they are. To his surprise at a very early stage of devilment the female plants have a noticeable potency to them. When it came time to harvest the 10 plants he realized that the female plants had seeds on them so he decided to save the seeds for next year to use for a new crop. Fortunately he had the plants in a none visible area of the yard, because people would take the plants if they saw them in that area. Of cause there are rules and regulation that Adam had to adhere to. Like not sell it, or give it away, or only have a certain amount of medical marijuana on hand. This was the first year that Adam tried growing his own medical marijuana so he would improve with every attempt to grow it. He soon felt better about the scars on his face and it would bother him less and less and he would learn to live with his disfigurement and accept it. He even found a woman that loves him for who he is and not just for what he looks like which she excepted.

The problems of injured war veterans, mental and physical can be astronomic and very a lot. Most of their problems last a life time. Many war veterans that have been injured are taking some sort of medication for whatever their particular problem. Hopefully in the future man will advance enough to cease all wars and live in peace with each other. This is one of many war veterans that is trying to adapt to a life changing situation that they are put in.

Ben B. suffered many INJURIES

Ben B. is 46 years old retired professional foot ball player that suffers from years of getting all kinds of injuries from broken bones to torn muscles and ligaments. All his past injuries have caught up with him and now he's paying the price with multiple sclerosis and rheumatoid arthritis and tendinitis. Ben also suffers from heavy steroid us that damaged his liver. His ailments have slowed him down considerably. Having been a famous figure and still well known is still popular. These days he is doing sports announcing on the radio and sometimes TV.

Five years prior he was in such poor physical way due to pain and discomfort, he was not able to work or travel. Ben would take all kinds of pain medication to deal with the pain of his multiple ailments. Throughout these years he tested different pain medications to see which ones would help his pain and still allow him to work. There are many different pain medications that should not be taken with other pain medications. Ben would choose one type of pain medication pills and medical marijuana to deal with his daily discomfort and pain. He says he's not as active as when he was younger and healthier but at least he can still work and be active in the sports field of announcing. Ben would have his good days and his bad days. Having multiple illnesses can effect certain areas separately or together. Ben said that he preferred to take medical marijuana than some other types of pain medication because there's no after effect symptoms and it doesn't clash with other pain medicines he's taking.

Bill S. suffered a War INJURY

Bill S. lost his legs in the Vietnam War and has been in a wheelchair for many years. He had stated that he had been using marijuana to combat heavy depression, sadness and self pithy after the end of the war. He also stated that if he did not use marijuana at that time he probably would have committed suicide. The marijuana seems to pick up his attitude and gave him other thoughts and alternatives that are positive. In doing this it seems to give him hope. These days Bill is doing very well with his photo lab service and is buying a new house to accommodate his needs.

WORD'S FOR THOUGHT II foil, chrysalis, eccentric, times, parlous, life, lightnings, sponge, proper, day, Hawaii, miscarriages, torrid, tredecim, live, checkmate, dream, mons, around, genetics, base, main, phobos, exchange, vibration, stalemate, cohort, fluorescent, centralize, you, pet, controversy, countenance, t thought, explicit, sun, intensive, if, noncontagious, thatch, biology, vorticosus, aqua, orphan, sitnalta, aerial, calcine, urgency, mutatio, sr, opportunity, denotation, ace, ring, accomplish, thought, prosperous, events, idea, medicinal, yellows, fever, future, illnesses, aeroplane, times, fons, low, energy, vaccinal, vortex, open, droop, infallible, fluent, all, day, arceo, arrival, circular, sign, ice, change, tempus, liberal, canoe, hew, astro, reheare, messages, counts, eat, nano, tyro, metronome, ellipse, felt, evolution, branchs, sandels, resumption, nondescript, pursue, variance, prejudicel, majestics, astroprojection, illuminate, or, manipulation, in, circulate, port, hieroglyphic, is, metus, distinct, bravado, article, discover, house, maze, fair, lexicon, elephant, tech, liberty, unwinds, lake, legislate, frozen, migrations, knife infant, aware, axial, hark, Haiti, identify, tsunamis, adventurous, laylines, infancy, boundless, goodhumored,.,

Depression

MEDICAL MARIJUANA HELPS FIGHT DEPRESSION:

Depression is quite common among women. Depression is a medical condition that affects 19 million Americans each year. Of those affected by depression, exerts estimate that women experience depression twice as men. In fact, over the course of a lifetime, nearly 1 in 4 women will experience a major depressive episode. And yet, only 1 in 5 women suffering from depression will get the medical treatment they need. If appears that the chances of a women becoming depressed may be greatest during peak childbearing years, roughly ages 25-44, but depression can strike a women at any age. Remember if you are a women with depression, you are not alone. The good news is help is available. Everyone gets sad sometimes, a brief blue mood, disappointments, grief after losing someone you love. Depression, though, is different. Depression is not just a case of the blues: depression is a serious medical illness often caused by an imbalance of chemicals in the brain. Much like diabetes, asthma, or heart disease, depression is a disease that requires medical treatment. Otherwise, if left untreated, depression can last months or in some cases, years. Compared with depressed men are more likely to experience: guilt, weight gain, anxiety, eating disorders, increased appetite, increased sleep. There are several signs and symptoms that can help a health care provider determine if a women has depression. If a woman you know has had at least 5 of the following symptoms for most of the day for more than 2 weeks, professional help should be sought. Feeling of sadness, depressed mood, and or irritability. Loss of interest or pleasure in activities, such as hobbies or spending time with family or friends. Changes in weight or appetite, in sleeping pattern or sleep too much or not being able to sleep at all. Feelings of guilt, hopelessness, or Worthlessness. Inability to concentrate, remember things, or make decisions. Constant fatigue or loss of energy, restlessness or decreased activity, recurrent thoughts of suicide or death.

Depression isn't something to be ashamed of, nor is a sign of a weak personality. People with depression cannot just snap out of it! No more than it would be possible for a person with diabetes or some other medical illness to just snap out of it! Some risk factors for depression in women are, family history of mood disorders in early reproductive years. Reproductive issues: for example, infertility, miscarriages, surgical menopause, postpartum depression. Loss of social support system (such as family, friends, or assisted living services) of threat of such a loss. There are 2 main treatments for depression counseling, also called psychotherapy, and medication. For some, women, either treatment may be enough, for others, the most effective therapy is a combination of the 2 treatments. Counseling, or psychotherapy, is often called talk therapy, and it comes in many forms. Antidepressant medication works by helping to improve the way certain chemicals in the brain work. Women experience depression about twice as often as men. Many hormonal factors may contribute to the increased rate of depression in women particularly such factors as menstrual cycle changes, pregnancy, miscarriage, postpartum period, pre- menopause and menopause. Many women also face additional stresses such as responsibilities both at work and home, single parenthood, and caring for aging parents.

PMS in Women

A recent NIMH study showed that in the case of severe premenstrual syndrome {PMS}, women with a preexisting vulnerability to PMS experienced relief from mood and physical symptoms when their sex hormones were suppressed. Shortly after the hormones were re-introduced, they again developed symptoms of PMS. Women without a history of PMS report no effects of the hormonal manipulation. Many women are also particularly vulnerable after the birth of a baby.

The hormonal and physical changes, as well as the added responsibility of a new life, can be factors that lead to postpartum depression in some women. While transient blue are common in new mothers, a full blown depression episode is not a normal occurrence and requires active intervention. Treatment by a sympathetic physician and the family's

207

emotional support for the new mother are prime considerations in aiding her to recover her physical and mental well-being and her ability to care for and enjoy the infant. In any given one year period, about 18.8 million American adults, suffer from a depressive illness. The economic cost for this disorder is high, but the cost in human suffering cannot be estimated. Depressive illness often interfere with normal functioning and cause pain and suffering but only to those who have a disorder, but also to those who care about them. Serious depression can destroy family life as well as the ill person. But much of this suffering is unnecessary. Most people with a depressive illness do not seek treatment, although the great majority even those whose depression is extremely severe can be helped. Thanks to years of fruitful research, there are now medications and psychosocial therapies such as cognitive behavioral, "talk", or interpersonal that ease the pain of depression. Unfortunately, many people do not recognize that depression is a treatable illness. If you feel that you or someone you care about is one of the many undiagnosed depressed people in this country. The information presented here may help you take the steps that may save your own or someone else's life. A depressive disorder is an illness that involves the body, mood, and thoughts. It affects the way a person eats and sleeps, the way one feels about oneself, and the way one thinks about things. A depressive disorder is not the same as a passing blue mood. It is not a sign of personal weakness or a condition that can be willed or wished away. People with a depressive illness cannot merely pull themselves together and get better. Without treatment, symptoms can last for weeks, months, or years. Appropriate treatment however, can help most people who suffer from depression. Depressive disorder comes in different forms, just as is the case with other illness such as heart disease . This pamphlet briefly describes three of the most common types of depressive disorder. However, within these types here are variations in the number of symptoms, their severity, and persistence. Major depression is manifested by a combination of symptoms that interfere with the ability to work, study, sleep, eat, and enjoy once pleasurable activities. Such a disabling episode of depression may occur only once but more commonly occurs several times in a lifetime. A less severe type of depression, dysthymia, involves long-term, chronic symptoms that do not disable, but keep one from functioning well or from feeling good.

Major Depression

Many people with dysthymia also experience major depressive episodes at some time in their lives. Another type of depression is bipolar disorder, also called manic depressive illness. Not nearly as prevalent as other forms of depressive disorder, bipolar disorder is characterized by cycling mood changes: severe highs {mania} and lows {depression}. Sometimes the mood switches are dramatic and rapid, but most often they are gradual. When in the depressed cycle, an individual can have any or all of the symptoms of a depressive disorder. When in the manic cycle, the individual may be overactive, over talkative, and have a great deal of energy. Mania often affects thinking, judgment, and social behavior in ways that cause serious problems and not everyone who is depressed or manic experience every symptom. Some people experience a few symptoms, some many. Severity of symptoms varies with individuals and also varies over time. Some symptoms of depression are: persistent sad, anxious, or 'empty' mood. Feelings of hopelessness, pessimism, feelings of guilt, Worthlessness, helplessness. Loss of interest or pleasure in hobbies and activities that were once enjoyed, including sex.

Decreased energy, fatigue, being slowed down. Difficulty concentrating, remembering, making decisions, insomnia, early morning awakening. Or oversleeping. Appetite and or weight loss or overeating and weight gain. Thoughts of death or suicide, suicide attempts, restlessness, irritability. Persistent physical symptoms that do not respond to treatment, such as headaches, digestive disorders, ad chronic pain. Some symptoms of mania are abnormal or excessive elation, unusual irritability, decreased need for sleep. Grandiose notions, increased talking. Racing thoughts, increased sexual desire. Markedly increased energy, poor judgment, inappropriate social behavior. Some types of depression run in families. Suggesting that a biological vulnerability can be inherited. This seems to be the case with bipolar disorder. Studies of families in which members of each generation

209

develop bipolar disorder found that those with the illness have a somewhat genetic makeup than those who do not get ill.

However, the reverse is not true. Not everybody with the genetic makeup that causes vulnerability to bipolar disorder will have the illness. Apparently additional factors, possibly stress at home, work, or school are involved in its onset. In some families, major depression also seems to occur, generation after generation. However, it can also occur in people who have no family history of depression. Whether inherited or not, major depressive disorder is often associated with changes in brain structures or brain function.

People who have low-self-esteem, who consistently view themselves and the world with pessimism or who are readily overwhelmed by stress, are prone to depression. Whether this represents a psychological predisposition or an early form of the illness is not clear. In recent years, researchers have shown that physical changes in the body can be accompanied by mental changes as well. Medical illnesses such as stroke, a heart attack, cancer. Parkinson's disease, Hormonal disorders can cause depressive illness, making the sick person apathetic and unwilling to care for his or her physical needs, thus prolonging the recovery period. Also a serious loss, difficult, relationship, financial problems, or any stressful changes in life patterns can trigger a depressive episode. Very often, a combination of genetic, psychological, and environmental factors is involved in the onset of a depressive disorder. Later episodes of illness typically are precipitated by only mild stresses, or none at all.

Although men are less likely to suffer from depression than women, three to four million men in the United States are affected by the illness. Men are likely to admit to depression and doctors are less likely to suspect it. The rate of suicide in men is four times that of women, though more women attempt it. In fact, after age 70, the rate of men's suicide rises, reaching a peak after age 85. Depression can also affect the physical health in men different from women. A new study shows that, although depression is associated with an increased risk of coronary heart disease in both men and women, only men suffer a high death rate.

Men's depression is often masked by alcohol or drugs, or by the socially acceptable habit of working excessively long hours. Depression typically shows up in men not as feeling hopeless and helpless, but as being irritable, angry and discouraged: hence, depression may be difficult to recognize as such in men. Encouragement and support from concerned family members can make a difference. In the workplace, employee assistance professional or worksite mental health programs can be of assistance in helping men understand and accept depression as a real illness that needs treatment.

Late Life Depression

Some people have the mistaken idea that it is normal for the elderly to feel depressed. On the contrary, most older people feel satisfied with their lives. Sometimes, though, when depression develops, it may be dismissed as a normal part of aging. Depression in the elderly, undiagnosed and untreated, cause needless suffering for the family and for the individual who could otherwise live a fruitful life. When he or she does go to the doctor, the symptoms described are usually physical, for the older person is often reluctant to discuss feelings of hopelessness, sadness, loss of interest in normally pleasurable activities, or extremely prolonged grief after a loss. Recognizing how depressive symptoms in older people are often missed, many health care professionals are learning to identify and treat the underlying depression.

They recognize that some symptoms may be side effects of medication the older person is taking for a physical problem, or they may be caused by a co-occurring illness. If a diagnosis of depression is made, treatment with medication and or psychotherapy will help the depressed person return to a happier, more fulfilling life. Recent research suggests that brief psychotherapy, talk therapies that help a person in day to day relationships or in learning to counter the distorted negative thinking that commonly accompanies depression is effective in reducing symptoms in short term depression in older persons who are medically ill. Psychotherapy is also useful in older patients who cannot or will not take medication.

Efficacy studies show that late-life depression can be treated with psychotherapy. Improved recognition and treatment of depression in late life will make those years more enjoyable and fulfilling for the depressed elderly person, the family and caretaker. Only in the past two decades has depression in children been taken very seriously. The depressed child may pretend to be sick, refuse to go to school, cling to a parent, or worry that the parent may die. Older children may sulk, get into trouble at school, be negative, grouchy, and feel misunderstood.

Childhood Depression

Because normal behaviors vary from one childhood stage to another, it can be difficult to tell whether a child is just going through a temporary 'phase' or is suffering from depression. Sometimes the patient become worried about how the child's behavior has changed, or a teacher mentions that your child doesn't seem to be himself. In such a case, if a visit to the child's pediatrician rules out physical symptoms, the doctor will probably suggest that the child be evaluated, preferably by a psychiatrist who specializes in he treatment of children. If treatment is needed, the doctor may suggest that another therapist, usually a social worker or a psychologist, provide therapy while the psychiatrist will oversee medication if it is needed. Parents should not be afraid to ask questions, what are the therapist's qualifications? What kind of therapy will the child have? Will the family as a whole participate in therapy? Will my child's therapy include an antidepressant/ If so, what might the side effects be? Among the medications being studied are antidepressants, some of which have been found to be effective in treating children with depression, if properly monitored by the child's physician. The first step to getting appropriate treatment for depression is a physical examination by a physician. Certain medications as well as some medical conditions such as a viral infection can cause the same symptoms as depression, and the physician should rule out these possibilities through examination, interview, and lab tests. If a physical cause for the depression is ruled out, a psychiatrist evaluation should be done, by the physician or by referral to a psychiatrist or psychologist. A good diagnostic evaluation will include a complete history of symptoms, when they started, how long they have lasted. How severe they are, whether the patient had them before and if so, whether the symptoms were treated and what treatment was given. The doctor should ask about alcohol and drug use, if the patient has thoughts about death or suicide. Further, a history should include questions about whether other family members have had a depressive illness and if treated what treatments they may have received and which were effective.

Manic Depressive Illness

Last, a diagnostic evaluation should include a mental status examination to determine if speech or thought patterns or memory have been affected, as sometimes happens in the case of a depressive or manic-depressive illness. Treatment choice will depend on the medications and psychotherapies that can be used to treat depressive disorders. Some people with milder forms may do well with psychotherapy alone. People with moderate to severe depression most often benefit from antidepressants. Most do best with combined treatment medication to gain relatively quick symptom relief and psychotherapy to learn more effective ways to deal; with life's problems, including depression. Depending on the patient's diagnosis and severity of symptoms, the therapist may prescribe medication and or one of the several forms of psychotherapy that have proven effective for depression.

Electroconvulsive therapy [ECT] is useful, particularly for individuals whose depression is severe or life threatening or who cannot take antidepressants medication. ECT often is effective in cases where antidepressant medications do not provide sufficient relief of symptoms, in recent years, ECT has been much improved. A muscle relaxant is given before treatment, which is done under brief anesthesia. Electrodes are placed at precise locations on the head to deliver electrical impulses. The stimulation causes a brief seizure within the brain. The person receiving ECT does not consciously experience the electrical stimulus. For full therapeutic benefit, at least several sessions of ECT typically given at the rate of three per week, are required.

There are several types of antidepressant medications used to treat depressive disorder. These include newer medications chiefly the selective serotonin reuptake inhibitors [SSRIs] the tricyclics, and the monoamine oxidase [MAOs]. The SSRIs and other newer medications that affect neurotransmitters such as dopamine or norepinephrine generally have fewer side effects than tricyclics. Sometimes the doctor will try a variety of antidepressants before finding the most effective medication or combination of medications. Sometimes the dosage must be increased to be effective. Although some improvements may be seen in the first few weeks, antidepressant medications must be taken regularly for 3 to 4 weeks in some cases, as many as 8 weeks before the full therapeutic effect occurs. Patients often are tempted to stop medication too soon. They may feel better and think they no longer need the medication. Or they may think the medication isn't helping at all. It is important to keep taking medication until it has a chance to work, though side effects may appear before antidepressant activity does.

Mood Stabilizing Medications

Once the individual is feeling better, it is important to continue the medication for 4 to 9 months to prevent a recurrence of the depression. Some medications must be stopped gradually to give the body time to adjust. Never stop taking an antidepressant without consulting the doctor for instructions on how to safely discontinue the medication. For individuals with bipolar disorder or chromic major depression, medication may have to be maintained indefinitely. Antidepressant drugs are not habit-forming. However, as is the case with any type of medication prescribed for more than a few days, antidepressants have to be carefully monitored to see if the correct dosage is being given. The doctor will check the dosage and its effectiveness regularly. For the small number of people for whom MAO inhibitors are the best treatment, it is necessary to avoid certain foods that contain high levels of tyramine, such as many cheeses, wines, and pickles, as well as medications such as decongestants. The interaction of tyramine with MAOs can bring on a hypertensive crisis, a sharp increase in blood pressure that can lead to a stroke. The doctor should furnish a complete list of prohibited foods that the patient should carry at all times. Other forms of antidepressants require no food restrictions. Medications of any kind prescribed, over the counter, or borrowed should never be mixed without consulting the doctor. Other health professionals who may prescribe a drug such as a dentist or other medical specialist should be told of the medications the patient is taking. Some drugs, although safe when taken alone can, if taken with others, cause severe and dangerous side effects. Some drugs like alcohol or street drugs, may reduce the effective of antidepressants and should be avoided. This includes wine, beer, and hard liquor. Some people who have not had a problem with alcohol use may be permitted by a doctor to use a modest amount of alcohol while taking one of the newer antidepressants. Antianxiety drugs or sedatives are not antidepressants. They are sometimes prescribed along with antidepressants, however, they are not effective when taken alone for a depressive disorder, stimulants, such as amphetamines are not effective antidepressants, but they are used occasionally under close supervision in medically ill depressed patients. Lithium has for many years been the treatment of choice for bipolar disorder, as it can be effective in smoothing out the mood swings common to this disorder. Its use must be carefully monitored, as the range between an effective dose and a toxic one is small. If a person has preexisting thyroid, kidney, or heart disorders or epilepsy, lithium may not be recommended. Fortunately, other medications have been found to be of benefit in controlling mood swings.

Among these are two mood-stabilizing anticonvulsants, carbamazepine {Tegretol} and valproate {Depakotel}. Both of these medications have gained wide acceptance in clinical practice and valproate has been approved by the Food and Drug Administration for first line treatment of acute mania. Other anticonvulsants that are being used now include lamotrigine (Lamictal) gabapentin {Neurontin}, and topiramate {Topamax} their role in the treatment hierarchy of bipolar disorder remains under study. Most people who have bipolar disorder take more than one medication for accompanying anxiety, depression, or insomnia. Finding the best possible combination of these medications is of utmost importance to the patient and requires close monitoring by the physician. Antidepressants

215

may cause mild and usually temporary side effects in some people. Typically these are annoying, but not serious. However, any unusual reactions or side effects or those that interfere with functioning should be reported to the doctor immediately. The most common side effects of tricyclic antidepressants, and ways to deal with them, are dry mouth, it is helpful to drink sips of water, chew sugarless gum, clean teeth daily. Constipation- bran cereals, prunes, fruit, and vegetables should be in the diet. Bladder problems- emptying the bladder may be troublesome, and the urine stream may not be as strong as usual, the doctor should be notified if there is marked difficulty or pain. Sexual problems, sexual functioning may change if worrisome, it should be discussed with the doctor. Blurred vision, this will pass soon and will not usually necessitate new glasses. Dizziness-rising from the bed or chair slowly is helpful, drowsiness as a daytime problem this usually passes soon. A person feeling drowsy or sedated should not drive or operate heavy equipment. The more sedating antidepressants are generally taken at bedtime to help sleep and minimize daytime drowsiness. The newer antidepressants have different types of side effects: headache-this will usually go away. Nausea-this is also temporary, but even when it occurs, it is transient after each dose.   Nervousness and insomnia-these may occur during the first few weeks.

Dosage reductions or time will usually resolve them. Agitation {feeling jittery} if this happens for the first time after the drug is taken and is more than transient, the doctor should be notified. Sexual problems- the doctor should be consulted if the problem is persistent or worrisome.

St. John's Wort

In the past few years, much interest has risen in the use of herbs in the treatment of both depression and anxiety. St. John's {Hypericum perforatum}, an herb used extensively in the treatment of mild to moderate depression in Europe, has recently aroused interest in the United States. St. John's Wort, an attractive bushy, low- growing plant covered with yellow flowers in summer, has been used for centuries in many folk and herbal remedies. Today in Germany, Hypericum is used in the treatment of depression more than any other antidepressant. However, the scientific studies that have been conducted on its use have been short term and have used several different doses. Because of the widespread interest in St. John's Wort, the National Institutes of Health (NIH) conducted a three year study sponsored by three NIH components, the National Institute of Mental Health, the National Center for Complementary and Alternative Medicine, and the Office of Dietary Supplements. The study was designed to include 336 patients with major depression randomly assigned to an 8-week trial with one-third of the patients receiving a uniform dose of St. John's Wort, another third a selective serotonin reuptake inhibitor commonly prescribed for depression and the final third a placebo. The study participants who responded positively were followed for an additional 18 weeks. After the 3-year study has been completed, results will be analyzed and published.

The Food and Drug Administration issued a public health advisory. It states that St. John's Wort appears to affect an important metabolic pathway that is used by many drugs prescribed to treat conditions such as heart disease, depression, seizures, certain cancers, and rejection of transplants. Therefore health care providers should alert their patients about these potential drug interactions. Any herbal supplement should be taken only after consultation with the doctor or other health care provider. Many forms of psychotherapy, including some short-term (10- 20 weeks) therapies, can help depressed individuals. "Talking" Therapies help patients gain insight into and resolve their problems through verbal exchange with the therapist, sometimes combined with homework assignments between sessions. " Behavioral' therapists help patients learn how to obtain more satisfaction and rewards through their own actions and how to unlearn the behavioral patterns that contribute to or result from their depression. Two of the short term psychotherapies that research has shown helpful for some forms of depression are interpersonal and cognitive, behavioral therapies.

Therapist for Depression

Interpersonal therapists focus on the patient's disturbed personal relationships that both cause and exacerbate or increase the depression. Cognitive behavioral therapists help patients change the negative styles of thinking and behaving often associated with depression. Psychodynamic therapies, which are sometimes used to treat depressed persons, focus on resolving the patient's conflicted feelings. These therapies are often reserved until the depressive symptoms are significantly improved. In general, severe depressive illnesses, particularly those that are recurrent. Will require medication along with or preceding, psychotherapy for the best outcome. How to help yourself if you are depressed. Depressive disorders makes one feel exhausted, Worthless, helpless and hopeless. Such negative thoughts and feelings make some people feel like giving up. It is important to realize that these negative views are part of the depression and typically do not accurately reflect the actual circumstances. Negative thinking fades as treatment begins to take effect. In the meantime, set realistic goals in light of the depression and assume a reasonable amount of responsibility. Break large tasks into small ones, set some priorities, and do what you can as you can. Try to be with other people and to confide in someone. It is usually better than being alone and secretive.

Family and Friends Can Help

Participate in activities that may make you feel better. Mild exercise, going to the movie, a ballgame, or participating in religious, social or other activities may help. Expect your mood to improve gradually not immediately, feeling better take. It is advisable to postpone important decisions until the depression has lifted. Before deciding to make a significant transition change jobs, get married or divorced. Discuss it with others who know you well and have a more objective view of your situation. People rarely snap out of a depression. But they can feel a little better, day by day. Remember positive thinking will replace the negative thinking that is part of the depression and will disappear as your depression responds to treatment. Let your family and friends help you.

How family and friends can help the depressed person. The most important thing anyone can do for the depressed person is to help him or her get an appropriate diagnosis and treatment. This may involve encouraging the individual to stay with treatment until symptoms begin to abate several weeks, or to seek different treatment if no improvement occurs. On occasion, it may require making an appointment and accompanying the depressed person to the doctor. It may also mean monitoring whether the depressed person is taking medication. The depressed person should be encouraged to obey the doctor's orders about the use of alcoholic products while on medication. The second most important thing is to offer emotional support. This involves understanding, patience, affection and encouragement. Engage the depressed person in conversation and listen carefully. Do not disparage feeling expressed, but point out realities and offer hope. Do not ignore remarks about suicide. Report them to the depressed person's therapist. Invite the depressed person for walks, outings, to the movies and other activities. Be gently insistent if your invitation is refused. Encourage participation in some activities that once gave pleasure. But do not push the depressed person to undertake too much too soon. The depressed person needs diversion and company, but too many demands can increase feelings of failure. Do not accuse the depressed person of faking illness or of laziness, or expert him or her to snap out of it.

Eventually with treatment, most people do get better. Keep that in mind, and keep reassuring the depressed person that with time and help he or she will feel better. If unsure where to go for help, check the Yellow Pages under mental health, health, social services, suicide prevention, crisis intervention services, hotlines, hospitals, or physicians for phone numbers and addresses. In times of crisis, the emergency room doctor at a hospital may be able to provide temporary help for an emotional problem, and will be able to tell you where and how to get further help.

Listed below are the types of people and places that will make a referral to or provide, diagnostic and treatment services. Family doctors, mental health specialists, such as psychiatrists and treatment services. Family doctors, mental health specialists. Such as psychiatrists, social workers, or mental health counselors, health maintenance organizations, community mental centers.

HIV and AIDS

HIV and AIDS

Research has enabled many men and women and young people living with human immunodeficiency virus (HIV) the virus that causes acquired immunodeficiency syndrome (AIDS) to lead fuller, more productive lives. As with other serious illness such as cancer, heart disease or stroke, however, HIV often can be accompanied by depression, an illness that can affect mind, mood, body and behavior. Treatment for depression, helps people manage both diseases. Thus enhancing survival and quality of life. Despite the enormous advances in brain research in the past 20 years depression often goes undiagnosed and untreated. Although as many as one in three persons with HIV may suffer from depression, the warning signs of depression are often misinterpreted.

People with HIV, their families and friends and even their physicians may assume that depressive symptoms are an inevitable reaction to being diagnosed with HIV but depression is a separate illness that can and should be treated. Even when a person is undergoing treatment for HIV or AIDS. Some of he symptoms of depression could be related to HIV, specific HIV related disorders, or medication side effects. However, a skilled health professional will recognize the symptoms of depression and inquire about their duration and severity, diagnose the disorder, and suggest appropriate treatment.

Depression results from abnormal functioning of the brain. The causes of depression are currently a matter of intense research. An interaction between genetic predisposition and life history appear to determine a person's level of risk. Episodes of depression may then triggered by stress, difficult life evens, side effects of medications, or the effects of HIV on the brain. Whatever its origins, depression can limit the energy needed to keep focused on staying healthy, and research shows that it may accelerate HIV's progression to AIDS.

AIDS was first reported in the United States in 1981 and has since become a major worldwide epidemic. AIDS is caused by the human immunodeficiency virus (HIV). By killing or damaging cells of the body's immune system, HIV progressively destroys the body's ability to fight infections and certain cancers. The terms AIDS applies to the most advanced stages of HIV infection. More than 700,00 cases of AIDS have been reported in the United States since 1981, and as many as 900,000 Americans may be infected with HIV. The epidemic is growing most rapidly among women and minority populations. HIV is spread most commonly by having sex with an infected partner.

The Effects of HIV

HIV also is spread through contact with infected blood, which frequently occurs among injection drug users who share needles or syringes contaminated with blood from someone infected with the virus. Women with HIV can transmit the virus to their babies during pregnancy, birth or breast-feeding. However if the mother takes the drug AZT during pregnancy, she can reduce significantly the chances that her baby will be infected with HIV. Many people do not develop any symptoms when they first become infected with HIV. Some people however have a flu-like illness within a month or two after exposure to the virus. More persistent or severe symptoms may not surface for a decade or more after HIV first enters the body in adults, or within two years in children born with HIV infection. This period of asymptomatic (without symptoms) infection is highly individual.

During the asymptomatic period, however, the virus is actively multiplying, infecting, and killing cells of the immune system, and people are highly infectious. As the immune system deteriorates a variety of complications start to take over. For many people, their first sign of infection is large lymph nodes or swollen glands that may be enlarged for more than three months. Other symptoms often experienced months to years before the onset of AIDS include, lack of energy, weight loss, frequent fevers and sweats, persistent or frequent yeast infections (oral or vaginal), persistent skin rashes or flaky skin, pelvic inflammatory disease in women that does not respond to treatment, short-term memory

221

loss. Many people are so debilitated by the symptoms of AIDS that they cannot hold steady employment or do household chores. Other people with AIDS may experience phases of intense life- threatening illness followed by phases in which they function normally. Because early HIV infection often cause no symptoms, a doctor or other health care worker usually can diagnose it by testing a person's blood for the presence of antibodies (disease-fighting proteins) to HIV. HIV antibodies generally do not reach levels in the blood which the doctor can see until one to three months following infection, and it may take the antibodies as long as six months to be produced in quantities large enough to show up in standard blood tests.

Therefore people exposed to the virus should get an HIV test within this time period. Over the past 10 years researchers have developed antiretroviral drugs to fight HIV infection and its associated infections and cancers.

Marijuana Used to Help AIDS Patients

Currently available drugs do not cure people of HIV infection or AIDS, however and they all have side effects that can be severe. Because no vaccine for HIV is available, the only way to prevent infection by the virus is to avoid behaviors that put a person at risk of infection, such as sharing needles and having unprotected sex.

While there are many different treatments for depression, they must be carefully chosen by a trained professional based on the circumstances of the person and family. Prescription antidepressant medications are generally well tolerated and save people with HIV. There are however, possible interactions among some monitoring. Specific types of psychotherapy, or talk therapy, can relieve depression. Some individuals with HIV attempt to treat their depression with herbal remedies. Using the herbal supplements of any kind should be discussed with a physician before they are tried. Medical marijuana can be taken with other medications for HIV. Scientists recently discovered that St. John's Wort, an herbal remedy sold over the counter and promoted as a treatment for mild depression, can have harmful interactions with other medications, including those prescribed for HIV.

In particular, St. John's Wort reduces blood levels of the protease inhibitor indinavir and probably the other protease inhibitor drugs as well. If taken together, the combination could allow the AIDS virus to rebound, perhaps in a drug resistant form. Treatment for depression in the context of HIV or AIDS should be managed by a mental health professional for example, a psychiatrist, or clinical social worker who is in close communication with the physician providing the HIV/ AIDS treatment.

Depression Caused By AIDS

This is especially important when antidepressant medication is prescribed, so that potentially harmful drug interactions can be avoided. In some cases, a mental health professional that specializes in treating individuals with depression and co-occurring physical illnesses such as HIV/ AIDS may be available. People with HIV/ AIDS who develop depression, as well as people in treatment for depression who subsequently contract HIV should make sure to tell any physician they visit about the full range of medications they are taking. Research has enabled many men, women, and young people with cancer to survive and to lead fuller, more productive lives, both while they are undergoing treatment, and afterward. As with other serious illnesses, such as HIV, heart disease or stroke, cancer can be accompanied by depression, which can affect mind, mood, body and behavior.

Treatment for depression helps people manage both diseases, thus enhancing survival and quality of life. About 9 million Americans of all ages are living with a current or past diagnosis of cancer. People who face a cancer diagnosis will experience many stresses and emotional upheavals. Fear of death, interruption of life plans, changes in body image and self-esteem, changes in social role, lifestyle, and medical bills are important issues to be faced. Still, not everyone with cancer becomes depressed.

Depression Caused By Cancer

Depression can exist before the diagnosis of cancer or may develop after the cancer is identified. While there is no evidence to support a causal role for depression in cancer, depression may impact the course of the disease and a person's ability to participate in treatment. Despite the enormous advances in brain research in the past 20 years, depression often goes undiagnosed and untreated. While studies generally indicate that about 25 percent of people with cancer have depression, only 2 percent of cancer patients in one study were receiving antidepressant medication.

Persons with cancer, their families and friends, and even their physicians and oncologists (physicians specializing in cancer treatment) may misinterpret depression's warning signs, mistaking them for inevitable accompaniments to cancer. Symptoms of depression may overlap with those of cancer and other physical illnesses. However skilled health professionals will recognize the symptoms of depression and inquire about their duration and severity, diagnose the disorder, and suggest appropriate treatment.

Depression results from abnormal functioning of the brain. The causes of depression are currently a matter of intense research. An interaction between genetic predisposition and life history appear to determine a person's level of risk. Episodes of depression may then triggered by stress, difficult life evens, side effects of medications, or other environmental factors. Whatever its origins, depression can limit the energy needed to keep focused on treatment for other disorder, such as cancer. Cancer can develop in any organ or tissue of the body. Normally cells grow and dived to produce more cells only when the body needs them. But sometimes cells keep dividing when new cells are not needed. These extra cells may form a mass of tissue, called a tumor. Tenors can be either benign (not cancerous) or malignant (cancerous).

Cells in malignant tumors are abnormal and divide without control or order, resulting in damage to the organs or tissues they invade. Cancer cells can break away from a malignant tumor and enter the bloodstream or the lymphatic system. This is how cancer spreads, or metastasizes, from the original cancer site to form new tumors in other organs. The original tumor, called the primary cancer or primary tumor, is usually named for the part of the body in which it begins. Cancer can cause a variety of symptoms. Some include, thickening or lump in the breast or any other part of the body. Obvious change in a wart or mole, a sore that does not heal, nagging cough or hoarseness, changes in bowel or bladder habits, indigestion or difficulty swallowing, unexplained changes in weight, unusual bleeding or discharge.

When these or other symptoms occur, they are not always caused by cancer. They may also be caused by infections, benign tumors, or other problems. It is important to see a doctor about any of these symptoms or about other physical changes. Only a doctor can make a diagnosis. One should not wait to feel pain, early cancer usually does not cause pain.

Treatment for cancer depends on the type of cancer, the size, the location, and stage of the disease, the person's general health, and other factors. People with cancer are often treated by a team of specialists, which may include a surgeon, radiation oncologist, medical oncologist, and others. Most cancers are treated with surgery, radiation therapy, chemotherapy, hormone therapy, or biological therapy. One treatment method or a combination of methods may be used depending on each person's situation.

At times it is taken for granted that cancer will induce depression, that depression is a normal part of dealing with cancer, or that depression cannot be alleviated for a person suffering from cancer. But these assumptions are false. Depression can be treated and should be treated even when a person is undergoing complicated regimens for cancer or other illnesses. Prescription antidepressant medications are generally well-tolerated and safe for people being treated for cancer.

There are, however, possible interactions among some medications and side effects that require careful monitoring. Therefore, people undergoing cancer in treatment for depression who subsequently develop cancer, should make the full range of medications they are taking. Specific types of psychotherapy, or talk therapy, also can relieve depression.

Use of herbal supplements of any kind should be discussed with a physician before they are tried. Treatment for depression in the context of cancer should be managed by a mental health professional who is in close communication with the physician providing the cancer treatment. This is especially important when antidepressant medication is needed or prescribed, so that potentially harmful drug interactions can be avoided. In some cases, a mental health professional that specializes in treating individuals with depression and co-occurring physical illnesses such as cancer may be available.

While there are many different treatments for depression, they must be carefully chosen by a trained professional based on the circumstances of the person and family. Recovery from depression takes time. Medications for depression can take several weeks to work and may need to be combined with ongoing psychotherapy. Not everyone responds to treatment in the same way. Prescriptions and dosing may need to be adjusted. No matter how advanced the cancer, however, the person does not have to suffer from depression. Treatment can be effective.

Other mental disorders, such as bipolar disorder (manic-depressive illness) and anxiety disorders, may occur in people with cancer, and they too can be effectively treated. Remember, depression is a treatable disorder of the brain. Depression can be treated in addition to whatever other illnesses a person might have, including cancer. If you think you may be depressed or know someone who is, don't lose hope. Seek help for the depression.

Lupus

Medicinal Marijuana Advocate Val C.

This Chapter is dedicated to Val C. a medical marijuana advocate that suffers from Lupus. And informing people about Systemic Lupus Erythematosus. Lupus is a type of immune system disorder known as an autoimmune disease. In autoimmune diseases, the body harms it's own healthy cells and tissues. This leads to inflammation and damage of various body tissues. Lupus can affect many parts of the body, including the joints, skin, kidneys, heart, lungs, blood vessels, and brain. Although people with the disease may have many different symptoms, some of the most common ones include extreme fatigue, painful or swollen joints (arthritis), unexplained fever, skin rashes, and kidney problems.

Lupus is also known as a rheumatic disease. The rheumatic diseases are a group of disorders that cause aches, pain, and stiffness in the joints, muscles, and bones. Symptoms of lupus can be controlled with appropriate treatment, and most people with disease can

226

lead active, healthy lives. At present there is no cure for lupus. However the symptoms of lupus can be controlled with appropriate treatment and most people with the disease can lead active, healthy lives. Lupus is characterized by periods of illness, called flares, and periods of wellness, or remission. Understanding how to prevent flare ups and how to treat them when they do occur helps people with lupus maintain better health. Intense research is underway and scientists funded by NH are continuing to make great strides in understanding the disease, which ultimately may lead to a cure. Two of the questions researchers are studying are who gets lupus and why? We know that many more women then men have lupus. Lupus is three times more common in black women than in white women and is also more common in women of Hispanic, Asian, Native American descent in addition, lupus can run in families, but the risk that a child or a brother or sister of a patient also will have lupus is still quite low. It is difficult to estimate how many people in the United States have the disease, because it's symptoms wary widely and it's onset is often hard to pinpoint. Although lupus is used as a broad term, there actually are several kinds of lupus. Systemic Lupus Erythematosus (SLE) which is the form of the disease that most people are referring to when they say lupus. The word systemic means the disease can affect many parts of the body. The symptoms of SLE may be mild or serious. Although SLE usually first affects people between the ages of 15 and 45 years old. It can occur in childhood or in later life as well.

Different Types of Lupus

Discoid Lupus Erythematosus primarily affects the skin. A red, rash may appear on the face, scalp, or elsewhere. The raised areas become thick and scaly. The rash may last for days or years and may recur. A small percentage of people with discoid lupus later develop SLE. Drugs induced lupus refers to a form of lupus caused by medication. It causes some symptoms similar to those of SLE (arthritis, rash, fever, and chest pain, but not kidney disease) that go away when the drug is stopped. Common medications that may cause drug induced lupus include hydralazine (Apresoline) procainamide (Procan, Pronestylo,

227

medthyldopa (Aldomet), quinidine (Quinaglute), isoniazid (INHO) and some antiseizure medications such as phenytoin (Dilantin) or carbamazepine (Tegretol).

Neonatal Lupus can affect some newborn babies of women with SLE or certain other immune system disorders. Babies with neonatal lupus may have a serious heart defect. Other affected babies may have a skin rash, liver abnormalities, or low blood counts. Physicians can now identify most at risk SLE patients, allowing for prompt treatment of the infant at birth. Neonatal lupus is very rare, and most infants of mothers with SLE are entirely healthy. Lupus is a complex disease whose cause is unknown. It is likely that there is no single cause but rather a combination of genetic, environmental, and possibly hormonal factors that work together to cause the disease. The exact cause may differ from one person to another. Scientists are making progress in understanding the causes of lupus, as described here. Research suggests that genetics plays an important role, however no specific lupus gene has been identified. Instead it appears that several genes may increase a person's susceptibility to the disease. The fact that lupus can run in families indicates that development of this disease has a genetic basis. In addition, studies of identical twins have shown that lupus is much more likely to affect both members of a pair of identical twins, who share the exact same set of genes, than two none identical twins or other siblings. Because the rick for identical twins is far less than 100 percent, however, scientists think that genes alone cannot account for who gets lupus. Other factors must also play a role. It is likely that there is no single cause but rather a combination of factors that work together to cause the disease. Some of the factors are studying include sunlight, stress certain drugs, and infections agents such as viruses. Even though a virus might trigger the disease in susceptible individuals, a person cannot catch lupus from someone else.   In lupus, the body's immune system doesn't work as it should. A healthy immune system produces antibodies, which are special proteins that help fight and destroy viruses, bacteria, and other foreign substances that invade the body.

The Affects of Lupus

In lupus the immune system produces antibodies against the body's health cells and tissues. These antibodies, called auto-antibodies contribute to the inflammation of various parts of the body, causing swelling, redness, heat, and pain, in addition, some auto-antibodies join with substances from the body's own cells or tissues to form molecules called immune complexes. A buildup of these immune complexes in the body also contributes to inflammation and tissue injury in people with lupus.

Researchers do not yet understand all of the factors that cause inflammation and tissue damage in lupus, and this is an active area of research. Each person's experience with lupus is different. Symptoms can range from mild to severe and may come and go over time. Common symptoms of lupus include extreme fatigue, painful or swollen joints, unexplained fever, and skin rashes. A characteristic skin rash may appear across the nose and cheeks the so called butterfly or malar rash. Other rashes occur elsewhere on the face and ears, upper arms, shoulders, chest, and hands. Other symptoms of lupus include chest pain, hair loss, sensitivity to the anemia (a decrease in red blood cells), and pale or purple fingers and toes from cold and stress. Some people also experience headaches, dizziness, depression, or seizures. New symptoms may continue to appear years after the initial diagnosis, and different symptoms can occur at different times. The following systems in the body also can be affected by lupus. Kidneys, inflammation of the kidneys(nephritis) can impair their ability to effectively get rid of waste products and other toxins from the body. Because the kidneys are so important to overall health, lupus in the kidneys generally requires intensive drug treatment to prevent permanent damage.

There is usually no pain associated with kidney involvement, although some patients may notice that their ankles swell. Most often the only indication of kidney disease is an abnormal urine test. Central nervous system ; in some patients lupus affects the brain or central nervous system. This can cause headaches, dizziness, memory disturbance, vision problems, stroke, or changes in behavior. Some of these symptoms, however, also can be caused by some treatments of lupus or by the emotional stress of dealing with the disease.

229

Blood vessels, blood vessels may become inflamed (vasculitis), affecting the way blood circulates through the body. The inflammation may be mild, and may not require treatment.

Blood; People with lupus may develop anemia or leucopenia (a decreased number of white blood cells). Lupus also may cause thrombocytopenia, a decreased number of platelets in the blood that contributes to an increased change of bleeding. Some people with lupus may have an increase in blood clots. Lungs; some people with lupus develop pleuritis, an inflammation of the lining of the chest cavity that causes chest pain, particularly with breathing. Patients with lupus also may get pneumonia. Heart; in some people with lupus, inflammation can occur in the arteries that supply blood to the heart(coronary vasculitis), the heart itself (myocarditis and endocarditis), or the membrane that surrounds it (pericarditis), causing chest pains or other symptoms. Diagnosing lupus can be difficult. It may take months or even years for doctors to piece together the symptoms to accurately diagnose this complex disease. Making a correct diagnosis of lupus requires knowledge and awareness on the part of the doctor and good communication on the part of the patient. Telling the doctor a complete, accurate medical history (For example, what health problems you have had and for how long) is critical to the process of diagnosis,. This information along with a physical examination and the results of laboratory tests, helps the doctor consider other disease that may mimic lupus, or determine if the patient truly has the disease.

Diagnosis of Lupus

Reaching a diagnosis may take time and occur gradually as new symptoms appear. No single test can determine whether a person has lupus, but several laboratory tests may help the doctor to make a diagnosis. The most useful tests identify certain blood autoantibodies often present in people with lupus. For example, the antinuclear antibody (ANA) test is commonly used to look for autoantibodies that react against components of the nucleus, or command center, of the patient's own cells. Many people with lupus test positive for ANA however some drugs, infections and other diseases also can cause a positive result. The ANA test simply provides another clue for the doctor to consider in making a diagnosis. There are also blood tests for individual types of autoantibodies that are more specific to people with lupus, although not all people with lupus test positive for these. These antibodies include anti DNA, anti-Sm, anti- RNP, anti- Ro (SSA) and anti-(SSB). The doctor may use these antibody tests to help make a diagnosis of lupus.

It may take months or even years for doctors to place together the symptoms to accurately diagnose this complex disease. Some tests are used less frequently but may be helpful if the cause of a person's symptoms remains unclear. The doctor may order a biopsy of the skin or kidneys if those body systems are affected. Some doctors may order a syphilis test because some lupus antibodies in the blood may cause the test to be falsely positive. A positive test does not mean that a patient has syphilis. Again, all these tests merely serve as tools to give the doctor clues and information in making a diagnosis. The doctor will look at the entire picture medical history, symptoms, and test results to determine if a person has lupus.

Other laboratory tests are used to monitor the progress of the disease once it has been diagnosed. A complete blood count (CBC), urinalysis, blood chemistries, and erythrocyte sedimentation rate (ESR) test can provide valuable information. (The ESR is measure of inflammation in the body It tests how quickly red cells drop to the bottom of a tube of unclotted blood). Another common test measures the blood level of a group of proteins called complement. People with lupus have low complement levels, especially during flares of the disease. These are some of the diagnostic tools for lupus. Medical history, complete physical examination, laboratory tests, complement blood count, Erythrocyte sedimentation rate (ESR) an elevated ESR indicates inflammation in he body, Urinalysis, blood chemistries, complement levels often low in people with lupus, especially during a flare. Antinuclear antibody test (ANA) positive in most lupus patients, but a positive ANA test can have other causes.

Other autoantibody tests; anti-DNA, anti- Sm, anti- RNP, anti- SSA, anti- La (SSB) one or more of these tests may be positive in some people with lupus. Syphilis test may be falsely positive in people with lupus, skin or kidney biopsy. Diagnosing and treating lupus is often a team effect between the patient and several types of health care professionals. A person can go his or her family doctor or internist, or can visit a rheumatologist. A rheumatologist is a doctor who specializes in arthritis and other diseases of the joints, bones, and muscles.

Treatment of Lupus

Clinical immunologists (doctors specializing in immune system disorders) may also treat people with lupus. As treatment progresses, other professionals often help. These may include nurses, psychologists, social workers, and specialists such as nephrologists (doctors who treat kidney disease), hematologists (doctors specializing in blood diseases), dermatologists (doctors specializing in disorders of the nervous system).

The range and effectiveness of treatments for lupus have increased dramatically, giving doctors more choices in how to treat the disease. It is important for the patient to work closely with the doctor and take an active role in treatment. Once lupus has been diagnosed, the doctor will develop a treatment plan based on the patient's age, gender, health, symptoms, and lifestyle. Treatment plans are tailored to the individual's needs and may change over time developing a treatment plan, the doctor has several goals: to prevent flares, to treat them when they do occur, and to minimize complications. The doctor and patient should reevaluate the plan regularly to ensure that it is effective as possible. Several types of drug treatments used to treat lupus. The treatment that the doctors chooses is based on the patient's individual symptoms and needs. For people with joint pain, fever, and swelling drugs that decrease inflammation, referred to as non-steroidal anti-inflammatory drugs (NSAIDS) are often used. While some NSAIDS are available over the counter, a doctor's prescription with other types of drugs to control pain, swelling, and fever. Even though some NSAIDS may be purchased without a prescription, it is important that they be taken under a doctor's direction because the dose for people with lupus may differ from the dose recommendations on the bottle.

Common side effects of NSAIDS, including those available over the counter, can include stomach upset, heartburn, diarrhea, and fluid retention. Some patients with lupus also develop liver and kidney inflammation while taking NSAIDS, making it especially important to stay in close contact with the doctor while taking these medications.

Some NSAINs used to treat lupus: Brand Name --Motrin, Advil, Naprosyn, Aleve, Clinoril, Voltaren, Feldene, Orudis, Dolobid, Relafen, Lodine, Daypro, Indocin.

Brand names included in this fact sheet are provided as examples only and their inclusion does not mean that these products are endorsed by the National Institutes of Health or any other Government agency. Also if a particular brand name is not mentioned, this does not mean or imply that the product is unsatisfactory. It can be dangerous to stop taking corticosteroids suddenly, so it is very important that the doctor and patient work together in changing the dose. Antimalarials are another type of drug commonly used to treat lupus. These were originally used to treat the symptoms of malaria, but doctors have found that they also are useful treatments for lupus. Exactly how antimalarials work in lupus is unclear, but scientists think that they may work by suppressing part of the immune response. Specific antimalaials used to treat lupus include hydrochlorquine (Plaquenil), chloroquine (Aralen), and they may be used alone or in combination with other grugs and generally are used to treat fatigue, joint pain, skin rashes and inflammation of he lungs. Research doctors have found that continuous treatment with antimalarials may prevent flares from recurring. Side effects of antimalarials can include stomach upset and extremely rarely, damage to the retina of the eye.

The mainstay of lupus treatment involves the use of corticosteroid hormones, such as prednisone (Deltasone), hydrocortisone, methylprednisolone (Medrol), and dexamethasone (Decadron, Hexadrol), Corticosteroids are related to cortisol, which is a natural anti-inflammatory hormone, they work by rapidly suppressing inflammation. Corticosteroids can be given by mouth, in creams applied to the skin, or by injection. Because they are potent drugs, the doctor will seek the lowest dose with the greatest benefit.

233

Short term side effects of corticosteroids include swelling, increased appetite, weight gain, and emotional ups and downs. These side effects generally stop when the drug is stopped. It can be dangerous to stop taking corticosteroids suddenly, so it is very important that the doctor and patient work together in changing the corticosteroid dose. Sometimes doctors give very large amounts of corticosteroid by vein (bolus or pulse therapy). With this treatment, the typical side effects are less likely and slow withdrawal is unnecessary.

Long term side effects of corticosteroids can include stretch marks on the skin, excessive hair growth, weakened or damaged bones, high blood pressure, damage to the arteries, high blood sugar, infections, and cataracts. Typically, the higher the dose of corticosteroids, the more severe the side effects. Also the longer they are taken, the greater the risk of side effects. Researchers are working to develop alternative strategies to limit or offset the use of corticosteroids. For example, corticosteroids may be used in combination with other less potent drugs, or the doctor may try to slowly decrease the dose once the disease in under control. People with lupus who are using corticosteroids should talk to their doctors about taking supplement calcium and vitamin D to reduce the risk of osteoporosis (weakened, fragile bones). Because some treatments may cause harmful side effects promptly report any new symptoms to the doctor.

For patients whose kidneys or central nervous systems are affected by lupus, a type of drug called an immunosuppressive may be used. Immunosuppressive, such as azathioprine (Imuran) and cyclophosphamide (Cyroxan), restrain the overactive immune system by blocking the production of others. These drugs may be given by mouth or by infusion (dripping the drug into the vein through a small tube). Side effects may include nausea, vomiting, hair loss, bladder problems, decreased fertility, and increased risk of cancer and infection. The risk for side effects increases with the length of treatment. As with other treatments for lupus, there is a risk of relapse after the immunosuppressive have been stopped.

In special circumstances patients may require stronger drugs to combat the symptoms of lupus. For patients who cannot take corticosteroids, A type of immunosuppressive drug called methotrexate (Folex, Mexate, Rheumatrex) may be used to help control the disease. Patients who have many body systems affected by the disease may receive intravenous gamma globulin Gammagard, Gammer, Gamine,) a blood protein that increases immunity and helps fight infection. Gamma globulin also may be used to control acute bleeding in patients with thrombocytopenia or to prepare a person with lupus for surgery. Working closely with the doctor helps ensure that treatment for lupus are as successful as possible. Because some treatments may cause harmful side effects, it is important to promptly report any new symptoms to the doctor.

It is also important not to stop or change treatment without talking to the doctor first. Because of the nature and cost of the medications used to treat lupus, their potentially serious side effects, and the lack of a cure, many patients seek other ways of treating the disease. Some alternative approaches that have been suggested include special diets, nutritional supplements, herbal supplements, fish oils, ointments and creams, chiropractic treatment, and homeopathy. Although these methods may not be harmful, it can be incorporated into to neglect regular health care or treatment of serious symptoms. Learning to recognize the warning signs of a flare can help the patient take steps toward it off or reduce its intensity. Despite the symptoms of lupus and the potential side effects of treatment. People with lupus can maintain a high quality of life overall. One key to managing lupus is to understand the disease and its impact.

Learning to recognize the warning signs of a flare up can help the patient take steps toward it off or reduce its intensity. Many people with lupus experience increased fatigue, pain, a rash, fever, stomach discomfort, headache, or dizziness just before a flare. Developing strategies to prevent flares can also be helped, such as limiting exposure to the sun (intense sun exposure triggers flares in some patients) and scheduling adequate rest and quiet times. It is also important for people with lupus to receive regular health care, instead of seeking help only when symptoms worsen. Having a medical exam and lab work on a regular basis allows the doctor to note any changes and may help predict flares.

The treatment plan, which is tailored to the individual's specific needs and circumstances, can be adjusted accordingly. If new symptoms are identified early, treatments may be more effective. Other concerns also can be addressed at regular checkups. The doctor can provide guidance about such issues as the use of sunscreens, stress reduction, and the importance of structured exercise and rest, as well as birth control and family planning. Because people with lupus can be more susceptible to infections, the doctor may recommend yearly influenza vaccinations for some patients. Warning signs of a flare: increased fatigue, pain, rash, fever, stomach discomfort, headache, dizziness. Preventing a flare: learn to recognize warning signals, maintain good communication with your doctor, set realistic goals and priorities, limit exposure to the sun, maintain a healthy, balanced diet, try to limit stress, schedule adequate rest and quiet times, participate in moderate exercise when possible, develop a support system. Patients who are well informed and participate actively in their own care experience less pain and make fewer visits to the doctor. People with lupus should receive regular preventive health care, such as gynecological and breast examinations. Regular dental care will help avoid potentially dangerous infections. If a person is taking corticosteroids or antimalarial medications, a yearly eye exam should be done to screen for treat eye problems. Staying healthy requires extra effect and care for people with lupus, so it becomes especially important to develop strategies for maintaining wellness. Wellness involves close attention to the body, mind, and sprit. One of the primary goals of wellness for people with lupus is coping with the stress of having a chronic disorder. Effective stress management varies from person to person. Some approaches that may help include exercise, relaxation techniques such as meditation, and setting priorities for spending time and energy. Developing and maintaining a good support system is also important. A professionals, community organizations, organized support groups. Participating in a support group can provide emotional help, boost self-esteem and morale, and help develop or improve coping skills, learning more about lupus may also help. Studies have shown that patients who are well informed and participate actively in their own care experience less pain, make fewer visits to the doctor, build self-confidence, and remain lore active. Tips for working with the doctor: find a doctor who will listen to and address your concerns. Provide compete, accurate medical information. Make a list of your questions and concerns in advance. Be honest and share your point of view with the doctor. Ask for clarification or further explanation if you need it. Talk to other members of the health care team, such as nurses, therapists,. Discuss any treatment changes with your doctor before making them.

Pregnancy for Women with Lupus

Thanks to research and careful treatment, more and more women with lupus can have successful pregnancies. Twenty years ago, women with lupus were counseled not to become pregnant because of the risk of a flare of the disease and an increased risk of miscarriage. Although a lupus pregnancy is still considered high risk, most women with carry their babies safely to the end of their pregnancy.

Experts disagree on the exact numbers, but 20 to 25 percent of lupus pregnancies end in miscarriage, compared to 10 to 15 percent of pregnancies in women without the disease. Pregnancy counseling and planning before pregnancy is important. Ideally, a woman should have no signs or symptoms of lupus and be taking no medications for at least 6 months before she becomes pregnant. Some women may experience a mild to moderate flare during or after their pregnancy: other do not. Pregnant women with lupus, especially those taking Corticosteroid. Also are more likely to develop high blood pressure, diabetes, hyperglycemia (high blood sugar), and kidney complications, so regular care and good nutrition during pregnancy are essential. It is also advisable to have access to a neonatal (newborn) intensive care until at the time of delivery in case the baby requires special medical attention. About 25 percent (one in four) of babies of women with lupus are born prematurely, but do not suffer from birth defects. It is important to consider treatment options during pregnancy. The women and her doctor must weigh the potential risks and benefits of each option to both mother and baby. Some drugs used to treat lupus should not be used at all during pregnancy because they may harm the baby or cause a miscarriage. A women with lupus who becomes pregnant needs to work closely with both her obstetrician and her lupus doctor. They can work together to evaluate her individual needs and circumstances.

The fear of miscarriage is very real for many pregnant women with lupus. The fear of miscarriage is very real for many pregnant women with lupus. Researchers have now identified two closely related lupus auto-antibodies, anti-cardiolipin antibody and lupus anticoagulant (together called the anti-phospholipids), that are associated with risk of miscarriage. One-third to one-half of women with lupus have these antibodies, which can be detected by blood tests. Identifying women with these antibodies early in the pregnancy may help doctors take steps to reduce the risk of miscarriage. Pregnant women who test positive for these antibodies and who have had previous miscarriages are generally treated with baby aspirin or the drug heparin throughout their pregnancy. In a small percentage of cases, babies of women who have specific antibodies called anti-Ro (SSA) and anti-La (SSB) have a symptoms of lupus such as a rash or low blood count. This is not the same as systemic lupus erythematosus and is almost always temporary. Most babies with symptoms of neonatal lupus need no treatment at all.

Identifying Genes

Identifying genes that play a role in the development of lupus is an active area of research. The current research of lupus is the focus of much research as scientists try to determine what causes the disease and how it can best be treated. Some of the questions they are working to answer include: Exactly who gets lupus, and why? Why are women more likely than men to have the disease? Why are there more cases of lupus in some racial and ethnic groups? What goes wrong in the immune system, and why? How can we correct the way the immune system functions once something goes wrong? What treatment approaches will work best to lesson or cure symptoms of lupus. To help answer these questions, scientists are developing new and better ways to study the disease. They are doing laboratory studies that compare various aspects of the immune system of people with lupus with those of other people both with and without lupus. They also use mice with disorders resembling lupus to explore how the immune system functions in the disease and to identify possible new therapies.

The National Institute of Arthritis and Musculoskeletal and Skin Disease (NIAMS), a component of the National Institutes of Health (NIAMS), funds many individual researchers across the United States who are stating lupus. To help scientists gain new knowledge, NIAMS also has established specialized centers of research devoted specifically to lupus research. In addition, NIAMS is funding several lupus registries that will gather medical information as well as blood and tissue samples from patients and their relatives. This will give researchers across the country access to information and materials they can use to help identify genes that determine susceptibility to the disease. Identifying genes that play a role in the development of lupus is an active area of research. For example, researchers suspect a genetic defect in a cellular process called apoptosis, or (programmed cell death) in people with lupus. Apoptosis allows the body to safely get rid of damaged or potentially harmful cells. If there is a problem in the apoptosis process, harmful cells may stay around and do damage to the body's own tissues. For example, in a mutant strain that develops a lupus like illness, one of the genes that controls apoptosis, called the fas gene, is defective. When it is replaced with a normal fas gens, the mice no longer develop signs of the disease. Scientists are studying what role genes involved in apoptosis may play in human disease development.

Researchers are also focusing on finding treatments for lupus. Studying genes for complement, a series of proteins in the blood that play an important part in the immune system, is another active area of lupus research. Complement acts as a backup for antibodies, helping them destroy foreign substances that invade the body. If there is a decrease in complement, the body is less able to fight or identify genes that predispose some people to the more serious complications of lupus, such as kidney disease, is producing significant findings. NIAMS supported researchers have identified a gene associated with an increased risk of lupus kidney disease in African Americans. Variations in this gene affect the immune system's ability to remove potentially harmful immune complexes from the body. Researchers are also making progress in identifying other genes that play a role in lupus.

Researchers also are studying other factors that may affect a person's susceptibility to lupus. For example, because lupus is more common in women then in men some researchers are investigating the role of hormones and other male- female differences in the development and course of the disease. Some promising area of research: identifying lupus susceptibility genes, searching for environmental agents that cause lupus, developing drugs or biologic agents that cure lupus. A current study funded by the NIMH is focusing on the safety and effectiveness of oral contraceptives (birth control pills) and hormone replacement therapy in women with lupus. Doctors have worried about the wisdom of prescribing oral contraceptives or estrogen replacement therapy for women with lupus because of a widely held view that estrogens can make the disease worse. However, recent limited data suggest these drugs may be safe for some women with lupus. Researchers hope this study will yield options for safe, effective methods of birth control for young women with lupus and enable postmenopausal women with lupus to benefit from estrogen replacement therapy.

Researchers are also focusing on finding better treatments for lupus. A primary goal of this research is to develop treatments that can effectively minimize the use of corticosteroids. Scientists are trying to identify combination therapies that may be more effective than single treatment approaches. Researchers are also interested in using male hormones, called androgens, as a possible treatment for the disease. Another goal is to improve the treatment and management of lupus in the kidneys and central nervous system. For example, a 20-year study support by NIAMS and NIH found that combining cyclophosphamide with prednisone helped delay or prevent kidney failure, a serious complication of lupus.

On the basis of new information about the disease process, scientists are using novel (biologic agents) to selectively block parts of the immune system. Developing and testing of these new drugs, which are based on compounds that occur naturally in the body, is an exciting and promising new area of lupus research. The hope is that these treatments not only will be effective but also will have fewer side effects. Other treatment options currently being explored include reconstructing the immune system by bone marrow transplantation. In the future, gene therapy also may play an important role in lupus treatment.

With research advances and a better understanding of lupus, the prognosis for people with lupus today is far brighter than it was even 20 years ago. It is possible to have lupus and remain active and involved with life, family, and work. As current research effects unfold, there is continued hope for new treatments: improvements in quality of life, and ultimately, a way to prevent or cure the disease. The research efforts of today may yield the answers of tomorrow, as scientists continue to unravel the mysteries of lupus.

Definitions

Adult ADD: Adult Attention Deficit Disorder.

Agitated Depression: is a psychiatric depression.

AIDS Disease: Acquired Immune Deficiency Syndrome.

Alzheimer's Disease: Dementia.

Anger Management: to manage one's anger or rage.

Ankylosing Spondylitis: affects the spinal column and joints.

Anorexia Nervosa: is the fear of gaining body weight.

Anxiety Disorder: feeling worry. Extreme apprehension.

Appetite Loss: not getting hungry.

Arthritis: Inflammation of the joints.

Atopic Dermatitis: is a skin inflammation that causes intense itching and discomfort.

Bipolar Disorder: a mood disorder.

Bronzed Diabetes: disease that takes too much iron from food that causes excess iron deposited in the liver, heart and other organs.

Bulimia Nervosa: is an eating disorder.

Cancer: the uncontrolled growth of abnormal cells in the body.

Carpal Tunnel Syndrome: compression of the median nerve.

Chronic Disease: a disease that persists over a long period. Swelling and dysfunction of the intestinal tract.

Collagen Disease: affects the bodies connective tissue or soft skeleton.

Communication Disorders: an impairment in the ability to receive, read, process, and comprehend concepts or verbal, non-verbal and graphic symbols systems.

Congenital Anomalies: a condition which is present at time of birth which varies from the standard presentation.

Crohn's Disease: a type of inflammatory bowel disease, (IBD).

Depression: (mood), a state of low mood and aversion to activity.

Diabetes: any disorder characterized by excessive urine excretion.

Digestive System Disorders: disease, diet, or emotional stress that causes a disruption in the digestive system.

Elevated Stress: increasing mental strain.

Endocrine Disorders: disorder in the Endocrine System, which is a network of glands that produce and release hormones that help control many important body functions.

Fibrocystic Breast Disease: manifest by multiple dense.

Fibromyalgia: disorder causing aches and tiredness. Breast masses and multiple tiny lumps. Masses enlarge and shrink with menstrual cycle.

Glaucoma: affects the optic nerve.

Gout: acute arthritis and inflammation of the joints.

Hemochromatosis: excess storage of iron in the body.

Herniated Disc: slipped disc.

Hypertension: is the elevation in systolic or diastolic blood pressure, (high blood pressure).

Hyperthyroidism: excessive thyroid hormones.

Immune Disorders: a dysfunction in the immune system

Infectious Disease: a transmissible or communicable disease comprised clinically evident illness resulting from infection.

Insomnia: difficulty in sleeping.

Leukemia: blood cancer.

Lou Gehrig's Disease: Amyotrophic lateral sclerosis (ALS), a debilitating disease also referred to as motor neurone disease.

Lupus Disease: a type of immune system disorder.

Mania: thought's are racing through their mind.

Menstrual Cramps: stomach pain or cramps.

Mood Swings: are controlled by the combination of thoughts and feelings which could put us in a good mood or a bad mood.

Multiple Sclerosis: (MS) the fatty myelin sheaths around the brain and spinal cord are damaged.

Muscular Rheumatism: See Fibromyalgia

Musculoskeletal Disorders: (MSD) can affect the body's muscles, joints, tendons, ligaments, and nerves.

Neoplasms: growth on tissue.

Neurasthenia: chronic fatigue.

Neurological Disorders: any disorder of the body's nervous system.

Osteoarthritis: form of arthritis.

Osteoporosis: bone disease.

Panic Disorder: an anxiety disorder, panic attacks.

Paranoid Schizoaffective Disorder: heavy fear.

Paranoid Schizophrenia: mental disorder.

Personality Neurosis Disorder: neurosis.

Phobias: an irrational or fear and dislike of something.

Polymyalgia Rheumatica: pain, stiffness in many muscles.

Polymyositis: an autoimmune inflammatory disease of the muscle that begins when white blood cells invade muscles.

Post Traumatic Stress Disorder: (PTSD) is when a person had experienced a traumatic event from the past.

Premenstrual Syndrome: (PMS) related to a woman's menstrual cycle.

Pseudogout: a rheumatologic.

Psoriatic Arthritis: a type of inflammatory arthritis.

Reiter Syndrome: it appears as a nonspecific urethritis. Arthritis and conjunctivitis.

Rheumatoid Arthritis: (RA) systemic inflammatory disorder.

Schizoaffective Disorder: mood disorder like bipolar, psychotic disorder.

Sciatica Pain: pain that goes down their leg through the sciatic nerve.

Scleroderma: thickening and hardening of the skin.

Scoliosis: curvature of the spine.

Sickle Cell Anemia: (SCA) autosomal recessive genetic blood disorder.

Skin Disorders: a disease or infection affecting the skill.

Sleep Disorders: (Somnipathy) is a mental disorder of the sleep patterns of a person.

Soft Tissue Rheumatism: autoimmune disease.

Spondyloarthropathy: a joint disease of the vertebral column.

Stiff Man Syndrome: a disorder that causes rigidity and stiffness of the axial musculature.

Stress: strain felt by someone, mental, emotional or physical strain.

Temporomandibular Joint Syndrome Disorder: joints in the jaw disorder.

Tendinitis: characterized by pain when the joint is moving.

Tennis Elbow: lateral elbow pain.

Tenosynovitis: pain when the joint is moving.

Tuberculosis: (TB) disease caused by various strain of mycobacteria.

Viral Meningitis: meningitis caused by viral infection.

Wounds or Injuries: traumatic injury, a body wound or shock produced by sudden physical injury, as from violence or accident.